A Busy Parent's Guide to Preventing Childhood Obesity.

Shawn Elliot

Holistic Nutritionist

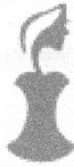

Table of Contents

Disclaimer   1

Preface   3

Part A: The Problem 7

    Chapter One: Health Risks 9

    Chapter Two: What Caused the Problem? 19

    Chapter Three: Perils of Processed Foods......................27

    Chapter Four: Impact of Sugar 43

    Chapter Five: Ditch the Diet Food 53

    Chapter Six: A Generation of Sitters..............................61

    Chapter Seven: Toxins and Chemicals............................71

        Bisphenol-A (BPA) 73

        Phthalates...74

        Atrazine 75

        Perfluorooctanoic acid (PFA)..76

        Synthetic Hormones 76

        Parabens...77

        Removing Toxins and Chemicals...................................78

    Chapter Eight: Negative Influences.................................81

    Chapter Nine: Our Relationship with Food.....................91

    Chapter Ten: Cravings and Habits 101

    Chapter Eleven: The Impact of Stress...........................107

    Chapter Twelve: Unexplained Weight Gain 115

Part B: The Solutions 121

    Chapter Thirteen: How Our Body Works 123

Fats 126

Carbohydrates 128

Protein 128

Water 132

Fibre 133

Immunity 134

Calories 136

Chapter Fourteen: Portion Sizes 141

Serving Size Summary 154

Daily Recommended Intake 157

Common Sources of Nutrients 158

Chapter Fifteen: Easy Swaps for Better Health 161

Chapter Sixteen: Saving Time and Money 171

Chapter Seventeen: Is Organic Really Necessary? 183

Chapter Eighteen: Change isn't Easy 195

Chapter Nineteen: Collaborating with your Doctor 207

Chapter Twenty: Emotional Support 215

Chapter Twenty-One: Are they Getting Enough Sleep? 225

Chapter Twenty-Two: Travelling Made Easier 231

Chapter Twenty-Three: A Final Word 239

Disclaimer

Disclaimer Notice: Please note the information contained within this document is for educational purposes only. Every attempt has been made to provide accurate, up-to-date, dependable, and complete information. Readers acknowledge that the author does not render medical advice and this book is not intended as a substitute for the medical advice of a physician. The reader should consult a physician concerning their child's health, particularly any symptoms requiring diagnosis or medical attention. By reading this document, the reader agrees that under no circumstances is the author responsible for any direct or indirect losses incurred due to the information contained within this document.

Preface

If you are looking for a book that contains multiple research studies, data, graphs, charts, complicated explanations, and terminology, then this is not the book for you. I know, as a parent, you are busy and do not have time to sit down and read a four-hundred-page book that explains how to create better health for your family. As a nutritionist, my clients would often ask me if I could create an easy-to-read book that provide facts and suggested solutions without needing a science or medical degree to understand the explanations, nor did they want to have to read multiple books to find the information they were looking for. I am going to be straightforward and honest. As a parent, there are some harsh realities that we face as parents if we want our kids to be healthy.

With more questions than answers, how is a busy parent like you able to help navigate this complex issue and help your child become healthy and happy with their body? How do you find the time to change your lifestyle when it is one thing you always seem to be lacking? How do you deal with the rising cost of healthy foods?

In every book I have read about childhood obesity, they blame the parent for feeding the child too much of the wrong food and not making them exercise enough. There are many variables about children's health that need to be considered, and blaming the parent has never made sense to me. I do not know any parent who has said 'gee, I think I will overfeed my child and make them obese, so they will have health problems for the rest of their life.' I know you want to protect your children and not make them sick; with this, in my opinion, blaming the parent is ridiculous, as it does not help anyone.

Many doctors simply recommend that their patients 'eat less and exercise more', yet this is oversimplified. Eating less of healthy foods is just as bad for the body as eating more unhealthy foods. So, it isn't about quantity as much as it is about quality. Some exercise is more effective at increasing your body's metabolism, so understanding the best kind of exercise for your situation is more beneficial.

If we want to point fingers and place blame, then what about the role of government in allowing foods that make our children sick remain available in the market? What about the advertising companies that are focused on marketing unhealthy food and drinks to our kids? What about the school boards that no longer support physical education classes or after school sports activities? What about the cost of living that forces us to work longer hours, leaving our children in the care of babysitters or at home alone in front of the television? And what about the rising cost of healthy food that forces us to purchase cheaper processed foods? Essentially, if you are looking for someone to blame for this obesity epidemic, you would have to blame everyone. There is no single person or element to blame and placing blame for such a complicated problem does not fix anything. Personally, I would rather focus on what we, as parents, can do to help our children become healthy right now.

Watching children suffer from obesity, bullying, and health issues breaks my heart. As a mother, I would do anything to help, and I believe other parents feel the same way. As parents, we want to take care of our children, but finding our way through the complicated issues of health care, school bureaucracy, healthy food availability and cost, access to safe play areas, and the hardest issue of all - time to do all the tasks that need to get done in a day, is almost impossible. We need simple tips we can implement immediately in our homes to help make our children healthier without being blamed for the problem.

In this book, you are going to find the answers to all of these questions. We will look at the changes in society and what caused this rapid change in the health of our children. And most importantly, I will provide suggestions that you can incorporate into your lifestyle to help improve the health and well-being of your children. Also, I will provide macronutrient information for various age groups as well as a holistic approach to health that includes better sleep, stress reduction, and emotional support.

This isn't a traditional 'nutrition' book, because I focus on macronutrients and changing behaviours rather than telling you about every single vitamin and mineral in various foods. Throughout the book, I have added in some fun recipes that your family may enjoy, which are simple to make, budget friendly and delicious.

Whether you are a single parent, blended family or have multiple children – this book will work for you because it provides strategies, not rules. This is not a 'diet' book for children as a balanced approach is healthier and more successful. My goal is to provide you with options for helping your child by giving you information on food groups, portion sizes, improving sleep, reducing stress and making exercise fun for the whole family. It is my hope that the information provided will benefit you and your children, so they can have the healthy body and future they deserve.

Part A: The Problem

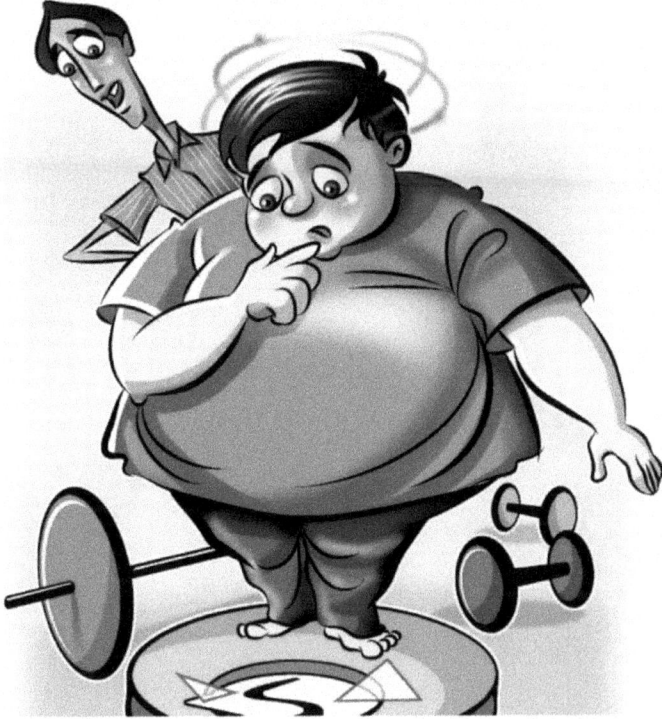

Chapter One: Health Risks

"Let food be thy medicine
thy medicine shall be they food"
-Hippocrates

1

We have been told that saying anything about a person's size is fat shaming and the subject is taboo. I would never want to body shame anyone, but is our political correctness killing our children? Have we normalized obesity?

As a holistic nutritionist and mother, I have seen firsthand the devastation obesity has on the physical and emotional health of children; children too overweight to run and play soccer with their friends, taunted and bullied by classmates, hating their own body and crying because they feel ugly and fat. Overweight children grow to become overweight adults and have to endure all of the disease and sickness that comes with this physical burden on their body.

When my daughter was given the diagnosis of being pre-diabetic, I was terrified. I knew the health risks associated with diabetes and wanted to do anything in my power to help her. She was an adult and understood that she needed to change but was still struggling to lose the weight. Our journey over the next few years gave me insight to weight loss resistance, hormonal imbalance, processed food addiction, adrenal fatigue and the lack of assistance by a medical system that is overburdened, underfunded and painfully slow.

It is important to understand that not all children who appear overweight are in any health danger. Many children grow out in weight, then up in height. They may have a larger bone structure compared to a smaller classmate or carry the 'baby fat' longer than others.

When you take your child to see their pediatrician to determine if they are in healthy weight, they will use the body mass index (BMI) chart that is standard in your geographical area to identify their weight percentile based on their age. I have an issue with this standardized chart because it does not take bone structure, muscle mass or whether the 'average' is actually a healthy weight into consideration.

Comparing a tall, big boned boy of German descent to a petite Asian girl doesn't make any sense. And as a greater number of people become overweight, the average weight goes up, which means our charts will reflect this. For example, in the 1960's, an average American ten-year-old boy weighed approximately seventy-five pounds, and in 2002, the average was eighty-five pounds. Our standardized charts need to be refined and updated to better reflect the health of the child, not just comparing their weight to other children their age.

As we discover whether or not our child has a weight issue, I want to point out that as a society, we have an unrealistic expectation of weight, especially for teenage girls who want to look like the models they see on magazines. Every woman I know wants to lose weight, whether they need to or not. We compare ourselves to models in magazines, actors on television and people on social media who have used filters to make themselves look different. All of us are unique, and we don't need to have a perfectly flat stomach, round booty and perky boobs to be beautiful. Our aim should be staying healthy, active and strong – not to fit the unrealistic ideal body type.

My point is to use your common sense about your child's weight and focus on health, rather than the numbers on the scale, which percentile they are at, or whether your daughter looks larger than models in a magazine or television.

The majority of overweight children grow up to be overweight adults, and we all know that being overweight contributes to a multitude of health issues, including type 2 diabetes, non-alcoholic fatty liver disease, heart disease, cancer, digestive issues, skeletal issues, and reduced longevity. Each of these illnesses can cause lifelong issues if diet and lifestyle are not changed. Let's take a quick look at some of the health risks we are facing.

Type 2 Diabetes

Type 2 diabetes was previously known as the 'Adult-Onset Diabetes' because it showed up in midlife; but now with the dramatic increase in the number of children who are being diagnosed, it is simply called type 2 diabetes. Insulin is a hormone created by our pancreas that allows the glucose in our blood to enter our body cells for energy. It acts like a key to the cell door that allows it to open and accept the glucose. Without glucose in the cells, we will develop type 2 diabetes, and if left untreated, we would die.

Insulin sensitivity or insulin resistance is when the cells become resistant to the insulin (they don't recognize it), which does not allow the insulin to open the cell door, causing the body to create more insulin to try and get the glucose into the cells. If our cells are unable to accept the insulin, the glucose will also continually increase in our blood. The higher the level of insulin in the body, the greater the risk of inflammation and disease.

According to an article in the National Library of Medicine (PMC 409943), most children with type 2 diabetes are obese or extremely obese at diagnosis. Being overweight has an adverse effect on glucose metabolism (how our body uses sugar), and obese children also have higher amounts of insulin in their blood than non-diabetic children.

Overweight children also have approximately forty percent lower insulin-stimulated glucose metabolism (the ability of the cells to use insulin) compared to non-obese children. In addition, the more visceral fat (the fat around the organs), the more insulin sensitivity in the child, which means they can't use the insulin they are creating because the cells are not recognizing it.

Risk factors for developing diabetes include family history, excess weight, sedentary lifestyle, high blood pressure, high cholesterol, and low-income status (due to inadequate access to fresh fruits, vegetables, and lean proteins). Studies and my own personal experience with clients have shown that type 2 diabetes can be reversed with a change in diet and lifestyle, which we will be discussing in future chapters.

Non-Alcoholic Fatty Liver

Non-alcoholic fatty liver disease is likely to be caused by a diet that is high in low-quality fats, such as deep-fried foods, processed meats, and high sugar content foods. Fatty liver negatively affects liver function which can contribute to diabetes, heart disease and kidney disease.

Our liver has five main functions which include filtration, digestion, metabolism and detoxification, protein synthesis and the storing of vitamins and minerals. It is the most important organ for detoxifying our body and maintaining good health. Harmful substances are filtered by the liver and excreted into our blood (to be removed by the kidneys) or bile which is a sticky yellow-green fluid made by the liver and stored in the gall bladder. Bile helps in digestion by breaking down fat into fatty acids so they may be absorbed through the digestive tract and separate harmful substances such as toxins and chemicals to be removed from our body as stool. Proteins are also created in the liver from the amino acids in our food which are necessary for cell structure and function. Vitamins and minerals are stored in the liver and then released into the blood stream.

As you can see, without a healthy liver, we will become sick and die. While twenty six percent of obese children have fatty liver disease (National Institute of Health, PM6440815), it can also be found in lean people who have poor diets. This disease can also be reversed with a change in diet and lifestyle.

Heart Disease

Heart disease (also called cardiovascular disease or CVD) was rarely seen in those under 50 years of age; but children in grade school are now being diagnosed and forced to take medication to prevent heart attack and stroke. Approximately seventy percent of obese children have at least one risk factor for CVD, and twenty five percent have two or more risk factors (National Library of Medicine, PMC 5575877). Again, this is being caused by a diet of processed foods, lack of fresh vegetables, high refined sugar foods, lack of exercise and insufficient sleep.

While I delve into this later on in the book, it is important to understand that processed foods lack the beneficial vitamins, minerals, phytonutrients and enzymes of natural whole foods. In addition, artificial food additives, colouring and preservatives put a huge burden on the liver and kidneys for detoxification and removal. Processed foods interfere with our gut microbiome which disrupts our digestion, absorption of nutrients and immunity. And these foods are high in saturated fats, processed sugar, salt and highly processed bleached flours which contribute to high cholesterol and coronary artery blockage.

Blocked arteries restrict blood flow and oxygen to the heart and may result in shortness of breath, fatigue, swelling in the legs or feet, chest pain, nausea, irregular heartbeat, stroke or heart attack.

Depending on the extent of the damage, it may be reversible through a change in diet and lifestyle, or at least prevent further damage to the arteries. Heart disease progresses slowly, so the earlier you can make changes, the better the long-term outcome.

Cancer

According to the Center for Disease Control and Prevention (CDC), being overweight or obese increases the risk of thirteen different types of cancer by seventeen percent and the risk of reoccurrence and death in some types of cancer by forty percent. While cancer may be caused by genetic disposition or environmental factors, we have also seen an increase in cancer among obese teenagers and young adults that has been attributed to lifestyle. As body fat increases, so do hormones that affect cell division, which increases the chances of this process going out of control and becoming cancerous. In addition, due to the Warburg effect (named after Dr. Otto Warburg), we know that glucose acts as a super food for cancer cells and reducing sugar intake can slow or reverse this disease.

While our genetics and most environmental exposure are beyond our control, we know a diet high in processed foods and sugar contributes to this phenomenon, and changing our diet and lifestyle will provide greater protection from many types of cancer. But how do we change our addiction to convenient processed foods in our extremely busy lives for a more natural approach? How do we stop our sugar addiction? Knowing the risk factors of obesity and its potential long-term problems is good information, but more importantly, how do we heal our children? How do we teach them how to have a healthy life?

Change is never easy, but it is vital we prevent childhood obesity and reverse the weight gain epidemic. Let's consider the changes in our society that have brought about this dramatic change in our children's weight and health and what can be done to reverse them.

Recipe: Breakfast Oatmeal

This easy-to-make breakfast takes minutes to be prepared and can be combined with any of your favourite berries.

Ingredients

Quick cooking oats (follow recipe on pkg for correct amounts)
1 Tbsp ground flaxseed
1 tsp cinnamon
Berries for topping

Follow the package directions and add in the cinnamon to the boiling water. Once cooked, sprinkle the ground flaxseed and stir in. Place in individual bowls and top with berries of your choice.

Tip:

Double the recipe and put half in a container in the fridge to make a healthy fruit cobbler tonight or tomorrow. Remove from fridge and place in either an oven or microwave container. Drizzle 1 tbsp maple syrup on the top and reheat (15 minutes at 350 or 2 minutes in the microwave). Add berries and reheat a few more minutes in the oven or another minute in the microwave. Serve in individual containers.

Chapter Two: What Caused the Problem?

"Children do learn what they live.
Then they grow up to live what they've learned."
-Dorothy Nolte

2

If we want to truly understand the problem of childhood obesity, we need to look back in time to when children were healthier and the changes that have occurred since then. In 1975, obesity was rare in children and affected less than three percent of the population. In the last thirty years, childhood obesity rates have tripled and now, according to Health Canada, over thirty percent of children aged 5 to 17 are obese in Canada and in the United States; one in six children is obese and one in three is overweight or obese (Harvard School of Public Health - Global Obesity Trends in Children). Think about this for a moment, this means that over fourteen million children in the United States are obese!

Childhood obesity and health related issues have risen dramatically, rates continue to climb, and for the first time in history, children are predicted to have a shorter lifespan than their parents. This generation isn't getting chronic diseases in old age but in adolescence, and is paying the price of convenience, rising food costs, and a generation addicted to technology.

The rapid increase in obesity began in the 1980's and has increased steadily ever since. But what happened in the 1980s that changed our society so dramatically?

Some people blame it on technology which has created a more sedentary lifestyle to the point where people never need to leave their homes. As we saw during the COVID-19 pandemic, children went to school, parents worked, paid the bills and did the grocery shopping online. We have become a generation of 'sitters' with chronic neck and shoulder pain from looking down at our phones, back and hip pain from sitting the majority of the day and chronic tendonitis in our fingers from texting and typing so much.

In addition to our personal technology creating a more sedentary lifestyle, manual labour practices began to change, declining from 68% of the workforce to 49%. When I was a kid, we had jobs on local farms doing haying, picking berries, mowing lawns, or other physical jobs. Now, with automation, most of these jobs have disappeared and many teenagers are standing behind the counter at a fast food restaurant, working as a barista or as a cashier.

An increase in the number of cars and public transportation have changed the way we get around, and fewer people are walking or riding bicycles than before. In the 1950's, it was normal to have one car per family. By 2005, the U.S. Census Bureau showed that twenty five percent of people had two cars, and in 2021, it increased to thirty seven percent. In my neighborhood, it is quite common to see a vehicle for each parent and teenager living in the home, which means less physical activity because they are not walking or riding bicycles.

This sedentary lifestyle means we are burning fewer calories each day, and we spend less time outside in the fresh air with access to sunlight and Vitamin D. Our bones are not as strong because proper bone density requires resistant exercise and/or weight bearing exercise, and without this we increase the risk of osteoporosis. Where children used to jump, run, roll, climb and play, now they sit in front of computers or televisions. According to the World Health Organization, "a sedentary lifestyle has serious implications for people's health and could be among the ten leading causes of death and disability. It increases all causes of mortality, double the risk of cardiovascular disease, diabetes, obesity, and increases the risk of colon cancer, high blood pressure, osteoporosis, depression and anxiety."

I've met people who blame the increase in childhood obesity on hormones and antibiotics added to meat and dairy products that disrupt our hormones, creating greater probability of weight gain. Growth hormones are given to animals to allow them to mature faster and gain weight in order to bulk up for slaughter. In an article by Leslie Brueckner in *Public Justice* (March 2014), it expresses their belief that these drugs make us fat. Amy Joy Lanou, PhD, Director of Human Nutrition at the Physicians Committee for Responsible Medicine in Washington, DC said that "people are eating meat from animals that have been given hormones and antibiotics to fatten them up. Those chemicals are concentrated in the animal's fat and passed on to whoever eats it." However, according to the Food and Drug Administration of the United States and Health Canada, growth hormones provided to animals pose a minimal threat to human health because they are absorbed by the intestines and liver of the animal.

There are also those who blame it on the changes in farming practices, from the smaller multi-crop farms to the mega mono crop farms which use genetically modified seeds and excessive use of pesticides and herbicides. These chemicals are believed to have depleted our soil which is no longer as rich with minerals as it was fifty years ago, which has impacted the nutrition of our food. Essentially, we are eating more food to obtain the same nutrients we require. At the same time, the food we are eating may contain trace amounts of the chemicals in the pesticides which can disrupt our hormones (called obesogens).

Due to increased mechanization and urbanization, pollution and global warming have also become hot topics. Air quality and climate change also directly affect us because toxins and chemicals can now be found in the air we breathe, the food we eat and the water we drink. According to the New York Health Foundation, Americans are exposed to as many as 80,000 chemicals currently used in the United States – few of which are adequately tested for their effects on health. Additional research hints that this toxic load can have a negative effect on our gut microbiome, unbalance our hormone levels and immune system.

As you can see, there are many ideas on what is to blame for the increase in obesity in our society, and I believe they are all a piece of the puzzle. But in my opinion, the biggest change that impacts our society today was the introduction of high fructose corn syrup, allowing for cheaper highly processed foods and the mass marketing of these foods into our daily diets.

Recipe: Baked sweet potato fries

Ingredients:

3 large orange fleshed sweet potatoes
2 tbsp extra virgin olive oil
1 tsp salt
1 to 2 tbsp spice (smoked paprika, chipotle powder, or
Cajun seasoning)
Parchment paper

Preheat oven to 450°F.

Peel the sweet potatoes and cut off the ends. Cut the potatoes in half lengthwise and then, if they are very long, in half crosswise. Cut each piece into 1/4 to 1/2-inch thick wedges.

Put the sweet potatoes into a large bowl and add the oil. Mix well to combine. Sprinkle with salt and spices of your choice.

Cover the baking sheet with parchment paper. Spread the sweet potatoes out in a single layer on the baking sheet.

Bake for 15 to 20 minutes. After the first 10 minutes, remove the baking sheet from the oven and use tongs to turn over all of the sweet potato pieces. Return to the oven and bake for another 5 to 10 minutes or until they are well browned.

If you want to make them more crispy, turn on the boiler on low for five minutes after baking, but watch carefully so they don't burn.

Chapter Three: Perils of Processed Foods

"Eating crappy food isn't a reward – it's a punishment"

-Drew Carey

3

High fructose corn syrup (HFCS) was introduced in the late 1970s as a low-cost alternative to beet and cane sugar. By the early 1980s, HFCS was introduced into soft drinks and processed foods, making these products cheaper, easier and faster to mass produce, which resulted in an inexpensive product for the consumer and the rapid expansion of the processed food market, changing the way we ate and our health.

Successful marketing targets these foods as 'cheap and convenient for busy parents' and 'fun and great taste' for children, which allows companies to sell them around the world at a staggering rate. For example, the Coca-Cola Company sells 1.9 billion servings a day worldwide, and the McDonalds Restaurant sells 550 million Big Macs each year in the US and 75 million in Canada.

Ultra-processed foods are filled with cosmetic additives, including artificial coloring, flavoring, thickeners, emulsifiers, gelling agents and preservatives to create a more satisfying and consistent food that lasts longer. Not only are these foods low in nutrients, which we learned earlier are essential for a healthy body, but these chemicals can disrupt our gut microbiome and lead to inflammation.

Our microbiome consist of trillions of microorganisms that contribute to a healthy immune and digestive system. These microorganisms help to digest our food, regulate our immune system, protect us against other bad bacteria that can cause illness, and produce vitamins, such as vitamin B12, thiamin, riboflavin and vitamin K.

Natural whole foods, such as bananas, oats and apples contain prebiotic foods that feed the good bacteria in our gut. Probiotic foods, such as kefir and sauerkraut, provide live bacteria which contribute to our microbiome. Highly processed foods do not provide the same prebiotic and probiotic benefits; they are believed to damage our microbiome balance by altering the ratio of 'good' to 'bad' bacteria, as well as killing healthy bacteria through the use of preservatives which are designed to destroy all bacteria to preserve the shelf life of the food.

Highly processed foods also contain high amounts of artificial flavouring, colouring, and sweeteners. To test just how damaging artificial ingredients and chemicals in our food can be on our bodies, researchers have studied how other animals react after ingesting similar foods and chemicals. One study in Georgia State University showed that emulsifiers alone can trigger obesity and gut health issues in mice when they consume these ingredients.

Food colouring in highly processed foods is used to create a more visually appealing food but has been shown to create health issues in some people. For example, a 2022 study on mice, published in the *Nature Communications,* found that frequent consumption of Allura Red (a very common synthetic colourant used in breakfast cereals, beverages and candies) may increase the chances of developing an irritable bowel disease, and long-term exposure may damage the gut lining. There are some who believe that artificial colours impact the brain receptors in children, affecting their behaviour, especially children with attention deficit hyperactivity disorder (ADHD). While some studies show a decrease in hyperactivity and ADHD behaviours when products containing food colouring is removed from the diet, more research is needed.

It is important to understand that even when approved for consumption in small increments, authorities often underestimate the amount of these chemical additives that will be ingested by our children. In addition, it is worth noting that studies are completed on each individual additive, to evaluate their individual effects on the body when consumed. However, this does not help when identifying how the interaction of these additives with each other in the human body can affect our overall health. At this time, there are no limits on the amount of these foods eaten by the public and most people do not understand the ingredients listed in processed foods. We trust our governments to protect us and have our best interest at heart when they approve products as safe to be sold as food. Yet, over time, we have seen chemicals and synthetic additives in highly processed foods that despite given approval as 'safe for human consumption, are not entirely good for our health.

Processed instant foods have become a massive part of our culture and day-to-day living. These convenient cheap foods have filled the gap in the life of a busy parent. I know many families who cook only with a microwave, a box or tin from the cupboard or frozen meal from the freezer; their refrigerators are empty of fresh fruit or vegetables, but their cupboards are full of boxes and canned goods. While processed foods may be cheaper and convenient, they are having a hugely negative effect on the mental and physical health of our children.

These foods are produced in factories, with low quality ingredients, and are full of additives. Its common ingredients are bleached white flour, high fructose corn syrup, processed white sugar, low quality oils and a list of chemicals that add flavour, texture, color and allow them to exist for years without decomposing.

Processed foods are often categorized into four groups, based on the amount of processing and ingredients: minimally processed/unprocessed, processed culinary ingredients, processed foods, and highly processed foods.

Minimally processed/unprocessed foods are items, such as fresh and frozen fruits and vegetables, dried beans, or nuts. There has been some processing from farm to table, but the effect is minimal as there are limited added ingredients. Processing is usually cleaning and removing inedible parts, fermentation, freezing, pasteurization, and refrigeration. These are the foods you want to eat the majority of the time.

Examples of minimally processed foods are:
- Fruits (fresh, frozen, dried)
- Vegetables (fresh, frozen)
- Beans (fresh, frozen, dried)
- Nuts (fresh, dried)
- Seeds (fresh, dried)
- Herbs (fresh, dried)
- Meat (fresh, frozen)
- Poultry (fresh, frozen)
- Seafood (fresh, frozen, canned)
- Oatmeal (with no added sugar)
- Quinoa
- Brown Rice
- Whole grains
- Milk

- Eggs

Processed culinary ingredients are used mainly for cooking or baking preparation and have been altered, but not in a way that is detrimental to our health. It's usually processed through pressing, milling, grinding or refining.

Examples of processed culinary ingredients are:
- Maple syrup
- Honey
- Salt
- Pepper
- Oils (natural oils only, no trans-fat oils)
- Starch
- Whole grain flour
- Spices

Processed foods are items which have added ingredients, such as sugar, salt, and oils. These should be reduced in our diet.

Examples of processed foods are:
- Bread
- Pastry
- Cheese
- Canned fruit
- Canned vegetables
- Tomato sauce (canned and jars)
- Meat products (ham, sausage, bacon, salami)
- Pasta

Highly processed foods contain very few ingredients from the first three categories, are meant to be super convenient, quick, low cost, and high in preservatives, fats, salts, sugar (in various forms), very refined grains, food coloring and flavouring. These are the foods we must avoid as much as possible.

Examples of highly processed foods are:

- Carbonated soft drinks, sugary coffee drinks, energy drinks, and fruit punch.
- Sweet or savory packaged snacks, such as chips, cookies, pretzels, and crackers.
- Sweetened breakfast cereals and instant oatmeal with added flavoring.
- Baking mixes, such as instant stuffing, cake, brownie, and cookie mixes.
- Reconstituted meat products, such as hot dogs, bologna, chicken fingers and fish sticks.
- Frozen and microwave meals.
- Powdered and packaged instant soups.
- Candies.
- Energy bars, protein bars and shakes.
- Meal replacement shakes and powders meant for weight loss.
- Boxed pasta products and instant pasta-based meals.
- Tinned/canned soups.
- Ice cream, sweetened yogurt, and dessert bars.
- Margarine and other ultra-processed spreads.

The biggest danger to our children's health is from highly processed foods and hundreds of studies have shown that a diet of these foods lead to increased rates of type 2 diabetes, colon cancer, bowel cancer, heart disease, arthritis, aging skin, tooth decay, fatty liver disease and other health issues.

Highly processed foods are calorie-dense, addicting, and quicker to digest. Our body does not burn as many calories digesting these foods (we burn relatively more calories digesting natural foods), leading to spikes in insulin. Spikes in insulin are usually followed by a persistent feeling of hunger and the need to eat again. In addition, these foods have fewer vitamins, minerals and fibre needed by our body to feel and stay healthy. Basically, highly processed foods offer little nutrition and an addictive quality that make us want to eat more.

Do you remember the Lays Chips commercial advertising 'I bet you can't eat just one,' which portrayed people struggling to just eat one of their chips? Well, they were right. Highly processed foods containing sugar and fat trigger dopamine (the feel good hormone), comparable to the need for nicotine or alcohol. The more often we eat these foods, the greater amount it takes to trigger that same level of dopamine. The more we eat, the sicker and unhappier we become. Nevertheless, because of the effect of dopamine, our bodies can easily become tricked, desiring these foods to make us feel better. It is a vicious cycle that has us trapped.

Highly processed carbohydrate foods (French fries, chips, cookies, cake, pretzels, muffins, instant pasta) are the most difficult to resist, restrict, and remove. These are the types of food that become our 'comfort food' during times of emotional stress. It feels like a dopamine fix is what will help us feel better, and our culture has become dependent on food to fill this need. Yet, in reality, there are a number of ways to ease our body's stress and also healthier, more rewarding food experiences besides a bag of chips.

As a teenager, I remember eating McCain-Deep and Delicious chocolate cake whenever one of my friends broke up with their boyfriend. We would commiserate with our friend and stuff ourselves with cake until our stomachs hurt. Eating that cake became a habit, and to this day, if I am upset, I still want that specific cake.

While fewer people have meat as a comfort food, highly processed meats are not any better as they contain a variety of additives that have been shown to be carcinogenic – or detrimental - to our bodies. Avoid feeding your child hot dogs, deli meats, bacon, beef jerky, and ham as there is strong evidence that they may cause cancer. The American Institute of Cancer Research and World Health Organization recommends avoiding these foods. In addition, eating processed meats has been associated with a higher risk of heart disease, high blood pressure, high cholesterol, and weight gain. If you love these foods, then this may be very difficult for you. When I suggested giving up bacon to my last client, she told me she would rather give up her husband than bacon. I get it, I love the smell of cooking bacon, but eating it every week is going to make your family sick. Learn to reduce the number of times you eat these kinds of food. For example, save the bacon for special occasions, such as a birthday or Christmas.

I have often been asked about turkey bacon and chicken wieners, whether these are healthier options and, sadly, no they are not. These alternatives still contain nitrates, high amounts of salt and saturated fats. Even veggie hot dogs are highly processed and should not be considered healthy. There is nitrate free turkey bacon on the market that can be a better option for the occasional meal, but as it is still very processed, I would not recommend it for your regular diet.

As highly processed foods have become the norm, we have become desensitized to the fact that we are no longer eating natural whole foods. Our grocery stores are full of these brightly coloured boxes, cans and bagged foods and we have come to expect and even demand these products in our diet. There are entire rows of boxed cereals, canned soups, pasta, candy, and crackers. Higher food costs and time constraints have also created a market for these instant foods and many families no longer cook from scratch but put together meals from processed foods.

In children, the effects of sugar, high salt and saturated fat are more pronounced as they have a lower body mass. Additionally, it has become normal for children to eat the same types of food as an adult and, often, the same quantity. When a six-year-old boy has a chocolate bar, compared to a forty-year-old man, for example, the impact is greater on the child. As children create eating habits from the food they are exposed to, the types of foods they eat, the amount of food eaten and when it is eaten, the risk of developing a diet of highly processed foods is increased. They get into the habit of poor eating, which gets worse as they age, bringing greater health risks.

Some children that eat predominantly processed foods no longer recognize various fruits or vegetables. I once made a comment to a young clerk at my local grocery store about how I would like to see more local apples rather than those imported from other countries. She responded with 'I don't think we grow apples in

Canada.' For your information, there are over forty different varieties of apples grown in Canada and are grown from coast to coast. According to Statistics Canada, in 2021/2022, Canada exported over 54,475 metric tonnes of apples to other countries. As processed foods are taking over our diet, knowledge of whole natural foods is declining.

In a study published in the *American Journal of Clinical Nutrition*, the eating habits of subjects were studied from 2001-2018, and the results clearly showed that eating whole natural foods declined throughout the period and highly processed foods increased, especially among lower socio-economic groups, college students and the elderly. The same group was re-evaluated in 2021 and the results demonstrated another increase in the consumption of highly processed foods and decrease in natural whole foods.

Highly processed foods are taking over our diets, but not providing good health. In another study from the American Institute for Cancer Research, over 100,000 subjects took part in a cancer research study and the results demonstrated that for every ten percent increase in the consumption of highly processed foods, the risk for cancer rose twelve percent.

The problem is, real food contains phytonutrients, vitamins, minerals, and fiber which are impossible to duplicate in artificially created products. Our bodies were not designed to live on highly processed foods, and the consumption of these foods are increasing each year while the consumption of vegetables, fruits and nuts decrease.

According to the Center for Disease Control, only ten percent of adults in the US maintain a sufficient intake of vegetables each year, and this rate is dropping yearly. The Heart and Stroke Foundation of Canada reports that seventy percent of children aged 8 to 12 years do not consume adequate servings of fruits and vegetables each day. A research article in *JAMA* by Lu Wang, PhD (August 10, 2021), has shown that over sixty percent of the calories in children aged 2 to 19 come from ultra-processed foods and contribute ninety percent of their sugar intake. While saving money and time are both ideal, our children's health has paid the price.

Despite these results, our society has not changed dietary habits, and the sale of processed foods continues to rise. The reality is these foods are difficult to remove from our diet because they are convenient, cheap, readily available and have become a part of our culture.

Not only are we eating fewer fruits and vegetables overall, but lower income families have less money to spend on groceries. And as food prices began to rise, cheaper processed foods began to fill the void. Single parent families also turned to processed foods for meals as they are faster and easier to prepare. It is no longer necessary to spend an hour making dinner, as it can be prepared in minutes, which allows the parent time for other activities.

Children can also prepare this type of food with the help of a microwave, creating a greater desire for processed foods. Let's be honest, children who are home alone while the parents are at work are much more likely to consume quick and easy processed foods rather than cutting up and cooking food from scratch.

As a busy parent you probably have to decide between time and convenience, cost or nutritional value when it comes to preparing the meals for your family. I can't give you more money on your pay cheque (I wish I could), but I can tell you how to create healthy meals that are quick and affordable and provide you easy food swaps and lifestyle changes to help you prevent obesity in your child.

Recipe: Green Smoothie

Green smoothies are a great after-school snack or breakfast on the run. You can change up these smoothies to add your favourite fruits and greens. Don't worry – you taste the fruit not the greens! Let older children help make these tasty treats.

Ingredients

1 apple or pear (for fibre)
1 cup frozen pineapple (or alternative)
1 cup frozen mango (or alternative)
1 cup frozen avocado or fresh avocado
1 Tbsp ground flaxseed or chia seeds (for healthy fats)
1 cup chopped lettuce (romaine or leafy not iceberg)
1 cup chopped spinach or kale
1 cup water (depending on size of blender)
Optional: celery, parsley, cilantro.

Blend everything together until smooth. Serve immediately or store in fridge or freezer.

Tips:

Fresh or frozen fruit or berries is fine but avoid seeds such as raspberries or blackberries or you will be chewing on them.

If you add greens to strawberry or blueberries, it will turn brown in colour (still tastes great though).

It can be frozen or kept in fridge for up to three days.

Chapter Four: Impact of Sugar

"Moderation. Small helpings. Sample a little bit of everything. These are the secrets of happiness and good health."

-Julia Child

4

Cocoa-Cola is a very popular drink in Mexico, and while I was living there, it was extremely common to see men taking a 2-litre bottle and a bag of tacos to work each day. I observed parents feeding Coca-Cola to their toddlers in baby bottles and giving it to young children daily. While they may have thought they were being kind to their kids, they were actually making them sick. Extensive exposure to the phosphoric acid in the soft drinks and high fructose corn syrup, which increases uric acid, has been associated with kidney disease and failure. Ten percent of children in Mexico are given soda from the time they are infants, and the country has a soaring rates of childhood obesity, diabetes, and kidney disease. Sitting in the waiting room of a medical clinic listening to a mother sob while the doctor tells her that her child has one of these illnesses is heartbreaking, and no parent should ever have to go through this.

We have all heard that sugar isn't good for us, but have you ever wondered why? After all, it comes from a plant, so it would be logical to assume it was fairly healthy for us. The biggest issue with sugar isn't the way it is processed, but the impact that it has on our body.

Sugar comes from either sugar beets or sugar cane. Sugar cane is harvested from the fields, washed and cut into shreds so huge rollers can press the sugar cane juice from the stalks. The cane juice is then clarified to remove solids and impurities, concentrated, crystalized and spun in a centrifuge to remove the liquid and produce raw golden sugar. It is then further processed through melting and filtering to remove the last of the remaining impurities (mostly molasses), crystalized again and then dried for packaging. The final result is 99.9% sucrose and approximately 390 calories per 100 gram serving.

If you read any articles on WebMD, Library of Medicine or a basic nutritional text, you will learn why excess processed sugar is considered harmful to our health. It is important to remember that sugar provides no nutritional value, and it is not a good source of energy, despite the short bursts of energy we think it gives us.

The negative health effects of processed sugar are:

- Tricks the body by turning off our leptin hormone which controls our appetite and turns on dopamine, the feel-good hormone, to make us want more of it.
- Too much added sugar can raise blood pressure, increase risk of chronic inflammation, which raises risk of heart disease.
- Our liver metabolizes it the same way as alcohol and converts it to fat. Excess intake can overload the liver, causing fatty liver disease.
- Raises blood sugar more rapidly than foods that are lower on the glycemic index, and extra insulin can thicken artery walls, making them stiff, which causes stress on the heart.
- Linked to atherosclerosis which are fatty artery clogging deposits.
- Increases risk of type 2 diabetes because it contributes to weight gain and increased body fat. Prolonged sugar consumption can make our body insulin resistant and burn out the pancreas.
- May increase the risk of certain cancers.
- Promotes tooth decay.
- Promotes inflammation which can raise risk of rheumatoid arthritis.

- Ages skin faster through a process called glycation.
- Associated with higher risk of acne as it can increase androgen secretion, oil production and inflammation.

As parents, we don't want to hurt our children and will usually give them sweets as a treat, but the effect on a small body is much greater than that of an adult because of their lower body mass index. Toddlers do not need sugar, ice cream, soft drinks, or other sweet treats. I know we often look forward to giving our child their first taste of ice cream or other treat food but put this off as long as possible because the sooner children are exposed to excess sugar, the harder it is to create healthy eating habits.

There are two ideas or trains of thought among nutritionists and dieticians about dessert and sweets: the first is that withholding them creates a bad relationship with food and can lead to binging or overeating. I understand their plight because when you tell yourself you cannot have something, then you crave it even more. If we eat this forbidden food, we feel guilty which can promote eating disorders and an unhealthy relationship with food. Remember, food is not 'good' or 'bad' and we are not 'good' or 'bad' if we eat it. Food is just nutrition, and it is there to contribute to our overall health.

The second belief is that due to the high caloric value of the common desserts and sweets (cake, pie, ice cream, candy), it is best to keep them to a minimum and for special occasions. My mother used to tell me, "You're sweet enough, you don't need sugar." Birthdays and Christmas were a time for cake, tarts, and sweets, but the other days were either fruit, berries or nothing. It is best to identify which special occasions or how often because if you don't clearly define this, these foods will slowly creep back into your diet on a regular basis.

To give you an idea how sweets and desserts can impact the total calories your child consumes, consider that one cup of chocolate ice cream has approximately 286 calories. So, if your child has one cup every night, they have consumed 8,580 calories in a month (a weight gain of 2.4 lbs) and 105,485 calories in a year (a weight gain of 30 lbs). If you replaced this cup of ice cream with a cup of strawberries, the calories change to 50 calories per cup, 1,500 calories in a month and only 18,000 calories in a year. Since the berries have essential nutrients and fibre which are used by the body, very little contributes to weight gain. Now, obviously, this is a very simplified example, but it demonstrates a valid point.

We have been brainwashed by the media that our children should be eating sugary foods, processed foods, fast foods, and instant foods. We see commercials of slender children at McDonalds, playing happily and eating their food, teenagers drinking Coca-Cola, sexy actors on television eating or drinking unhealthy foods, and we start to believe this is normal. We watch television and are exposed to constant food commercials for cereals, soda, fast food restaurants and processed foods, and this creates a subconscious impact on our food choices.

I remember the Kool-Aid commercials showing happy kids at a picnic or party, drinking with the Kool-Aid Man (he looked like a pitcher of Kool-Aid with a happy face and arms and legs) and having fun. I begged my mom to purchase these products because I wanted what they had (or at least what I thought they had). For your information, the Kool Aid mix called for six cups of sugar in a jug of water! It also contained artificial coloring ingredients that have since been banned in many countries.

It is time to change our culture and habits from a focus on processed sugar and ultra-processed food to natural foods that provide health, not disease. I believe that advertising laws need to be changed to prevent companies from promoting unhealthy foods to children and teenagers. I also believe that government policies should be changed from allowing foods that are deemed 'safe for human consumption' but don't provide any health benefits to promoting natural healthy foods. While advertising laws, corporations and changing government policy are beyond the scope of this book, as parents, we can control the media our children are exposed to and what we choose to purchase.

If your children are eating highly caloric desserts every night, removing dessert may be in order. You may start by swapping high processed sugar desserts for fruit or berries. They are still sweet but provide essential nutrients. Canned fruit is high in sugar and the fibre has broken down as a result of the processing involved in preserving and canning the fruit. Fiber plays a key role in helping the body feel full and it also slows the absorption of the glucose and rush of insulin. So, fresh or frozen fruits and berries are the best alternative for sweets. After switching them to a healthier dessert, you can decide if you want to cut back on eating desserts overall.

Another way to reduce processed sugar in your child's diet is to learn to read the labels on the products you purchase. Aim to have no more than six teaspoons of sugar (25 grams) a day. According to WebMD, there are 61 names for sugar. Therefore, we need to learn the most common ones that are used by manufacturers such as:

- Evaporated cane juice
- Fruit juice concentrate
- Brown rice syrup
- Malt syrup
- Corn syrup
- High fructose corn syrup
- Barley malt
- Galactose
- Glucose
- Sucrose

As parents, we know that candy and desserts are high in sugar, but did you know that a lot of other popular foods are also high in sugar?

Example:

- Boxed breakfast cereals
- Flavoured milk
- Sports and energy drinks
- Soda, lemonade, fruit drinks, fruit punch
- Energy bars
- Flavoured yogurt
- Jam, jelly, and peanut butter (with molasses)
- Baked goods
- Granola
- Ketchup, barbeque sauce, salad dressing
- Baked beans

By reading labels and swapping out foods that are high in sugar for whole natural foods, you can greatly decrease the amount they are eating or drinking. If you can't or don't want to cut out a food completely, try reducing the serving size of your child's favourite sugary treat and serve it less often, which can help to lower the amount of sugar they are eating.

Recipe: Grilled Bruschetta Chicken

Ingredients:

4 oz chicken breast (skinless)
¾ tomato (medium diced)
2 tbsp. red onion (finely diced)
½ garlic (cloves, minced)
1 tbsp basil leaves (chopped)
¾ tbsp extra virgin olive oil
¾ tsp balsamic vinegar

Preheat grill to medium and cook chicken 10 to 15 minutes per side until cooked thoroughly or bake in oven at 350 degrees for 30 minutes.

In a small bowl, combine tomatoes, red onion, garlic, basil, olive oil and balsamic vinegar. Add salt and pepper to taste.

Serve chicken breast topped with the bruschetta mix.

Tips:

Serve on grilled or roasted vegetables, bed of leafy greens, quinoa or brown rice.

Double the recipe and use leftovers for topping on baked potato or baked fish.

Chapter Five: Ditch the Diet Food

"The food you eat can either be the safest and most powerful form of medicine or the slowest form of poison"

-Ann Wigmore

5

Let's talk a little bit about *diet* snacks. There are a lot of snacks marketed to children that are labelled as 'healthy' or 'low fat' that are not worth the package they are in. Labelling laws allow manufacturers to use words like *healthy, low fat, low in sugar,* but it doesn't mean they are healthy. For example, a product may be low in sugar but extremely high in salt or fat. They also put pictures of whole fruits, trees, sunshine and use words like *wholesome, natural*, and *made from real fruit,* which is misleading. These words are not regulated and can make us think we are eating a healthy item while, in actuality, we are not.

I remember when 'diet cookies' came on the market. The first ones I saw were tiny little chocolate chip cookies in small one hundred calorie packages and of course, my daughter begged me to buy them for her lunches (who says advertising doesn't work?). Pretty soon, you could get anything in these one hundred calorie packages: chips, crackers, candy, and cookies. She was not eating any better, instead she was just eating smaller portions of terrible food, and often several packages because she was still hungry after eating only one.

Natural whole foods are always better, but if you need a packaged snack, look at the ingredients on the package. The first ingredient is always the largest percentage of the product, then the second and so on. If the first three ingredients include sugar (remember there are over seventy different names for sugar), salt, or a fat such as hydrogenated or partially hydrogenated vegetable oil, palm oil or palm kernel, I avoid the product. Processed snack foods are almost always made with a lot of preservatives, processed white flour, artificial flavouring and colouring, sugar, fat, and salt which are much harder on your child's body.

Along with *diet* snack foods, you also need to remove the ultra-processed *diet* foods from their eating habits. Crazy fad diets have been around since the 1930s, but it was in the late 1980s that highly processed *diet* foods really became popular. Every food manufacturer and restaurant got onto the low-fat diet trend that was believed to be the secret weapon against the rise of obesity and heart disease. Frozen diet meals, such as Lean Cuisine, Hungry Man, Children Cuisine, and Swanson TV dinners, became very popular, and even McDonald's had a McLean Deluxe Burger.

The low-fat diet that was promoted by the government and every food manufacturer in the 1980s taught us one thing – low fat does not make us healthier. We need healthy fats to absorb fat soluble vitamins, create cholesterol (yes, we need some to create our hormones), slow digestion, and aid in feeling full. What we don't need is poor-quality fats and high amounts of sugar and HFCS in our diet.

After the low-fat fiasco, the next diet style which became very popular was the 'sugar free' diet foods which sounds great in theory, but the problem is that the sugar in these highly processed foods became replaced by HFCS, low quality fats, artificial sweeteners, and salt. Consumers expect to have the same taste and texture in foods and removing the sugar meant producers needed to replace it with something that would keep bringing buyers back. By replacing sugar with HFCS or artificial sweeteners, manufacturers could advertise a food as *sugar free* which consumers believed was healthier for them, but little did they know they were trading sugar in for something just as bad or worse.

When you see words such as *no sugar added* or *contains real fruit,* you may think these are healthier alternatives for your child. *No added sugar* means they did not add sugar while processing, but it may still contain natural sugars, artificial sweeteners, or other additives to provide the taste and texture that is pleasing to us. The *contains real fruit* label means very little as it could contain as little as one percent real fruit that has undergone a massive amount of processing and now has no nutritional value. Do not believe the advertising of highly processed foods as your optimal health is not their goal. They are in business to make money, not to keep you healthy.

Diet soda sweetened with aspartame is not any better than soda with sugar. In fact, it may be worse. The World Health Organization (WHO) recently labelled aspartame as a potential cause of cancer. However, the FDA has argued that aspartame is safe. Whether you choose to believe the FDA or WHO, artificial sweeteners do not activate the same hormones in the brain that tell us our sweet craving has been satisfied, often causing people to drink more of the product.

Artificial sweeteners have been suspected (but not proven) of hormonal imbalance, cellular inflammation, liver damage, migraines, depression, irritable bowel syndrome, lowering the metabolism and cancers. There have been cases where a sweetener has been removed from the market years later because of these issues. Whether or not you choose to believe the various studies indicating that an artificial sweetener is safe, unsafe or may cause disease, replacing these foods with more natural options will provide your child with better health.

Children are growing and need whole natural foods that provide the essential vitamins, minerals, fiber, protein, phytonutrients, and water they require. Diet or low-calorie foods may not help your child lose weight but may encourage them to eat more of the processed food because they think it is lower in calories so they can have more.

These *diet* foods are not any healthier for your child. In fact, they may be causing more harm than good. By eliminating or at least significantly reducing *diet* foods, you can focus on providing whole natural foods that will fill them up without causing health issues and provide them the essential nutrients they need to be healthy. You will also be teaching them the right path to follow by not promoting a life of constant dieting and ill health.

Never give your child a weight loss supplement, such as Xentermine, OxiPhex, Garcinia Extract, CapsiMax, etc., without first discussing it with your doctor. Many diet supplements contain ingredients that can seriously harm and even kill a child. Diet supplements are not regulated in the same manner as medication and are created for an adult weight. If you choose to use a diet supplement for yourself, treat it like a medicine and be sure to keep it locked away from children as they may try your supplement for themselves and become very ill.

Recipe: Chicken Soup

Ingredients:

  1 tablespoon olive oil
  1 1/2 pounds uncooked boneless skinless chicken
  breast, diced
  1/2 tablespoon olive oil
  1 onion, (red or white) chopped
  2 garlic cloves (peeled and minced)
  2 large carrots, sliced
  3 cups diced potatoes
  2 cups chopped broccoli florets
  1 teaspoon dried thyme
  4 cups low sodium chicken broth
  1/2 teaspoon salt
  Freshly ground black pepper
  1 cup frozen peas

Place a large pot over medium high heat. Add in olive oil, then diced chicken breast. Cook chicken for 4-6 minutes or until thoroughly cooked and no longer pink. Remove chicken from pot and transfer to a large bowl; set aside for later.

In the same pot, add in olive oil, chopped onion, garlic, sliced carrots, diced potatoes, diced broccoli and thyme. Sauté for a few minutes until onion begins to soften, then add in chicken broth, salt, and pepper. Allow mixture to simmer uncovered for 10 minutes or until potatoes are fork tender.

Stir in cooked chicken and frozen peas. Allow mixture to simmer for 5-10 more minutes.

Taste and add salt and pepper, if necessary.

Chapter Six: A Generation of Sitters

"Exercise is the key not only to physical health but to peace of mind."

-Nelson Mandela

6

While our children are eating more processed foods that are causing weight gain, they are not active due to the lack of a safe space for play, more time on cell phones, computers and watching television and a decrease in participation levels in physical education classes at school.

When children arrive home from school to an empty house, as parents, we encourage them to stay inside where they are safe which also encourages them to be more sedentary. They come home, have a snack, and watch television, play on a computer or with video games until we arrive home. This sedentary routine is causing issues because the more they engage in those activities, the higher the risk for obesity, sleep problems, neck issues, poor vision, and tendonitis of the fingers and thumbs.

Kids need one hour of exercise or movement a day, but it does not need to be continuous. For example, they may have thirty minutes at lunch time and another thirty minutes in the evening. Their exercise doesn't have to be formal but can be anything that gets them moving, such as walking the dog, raking leaves, playing basketball, or a game of tag.

In order to determine if they are getting enough exercise, do an assessment of your child's activity level and how much screen time they have each day. How often are they outside playing? What do they do with their friends? Are they sitting around playing video games or running around the neighborhood? Are they involved in sports? And finally, are they active every day?

If your child is not getting enough exercise, start by limiting screen time (computer, phone, television, and video games), unless they require it for homework. I want to warn you in advance that they will not be happy about this (that may be the understatement of the year) but stick to your decision. The provincial government of British Columbia recommends limiting the amount of screen time to no more than one hour for children between the age of two and twelve, and two hours (including homework time) for children aged thirteen to eighteen. You may need to gradually decrease the amount of time in order to avoid issues with your child. Our kids are as addicted to their electronics as we are.

Limiting screen time will have several benefits. Television is especially troublesome as it is full of advertisements for processed foods and drinks that will encourage unhealthy behaviors, so less screen time means they are exposed to fewer advertisements. Less time on cell phones and computers means less access to social media and the all the pressures that can put on a young person. And if they aren't sitting playing video games, they can play games that require their imagination, flexibility, build strength and teamwork skills.

Encourage them to get outside to play and be physically active. In my experience, telling a child to go outside and play may result in them sitting outside doing nothing until they get in the habit of being active, which means you are going to need to play with them by teaching them to play a sport or going for a walk with them or some other activity. Not only will you get your exercise in, but you get to spend some quality time with your child.

When my daughter was a teenager, we started going for a walk together in the evening and I found that she would open up to me about things in her life that she never did before. Perhaps it was because we had such a peaceful activity with no distractions. But the conversations with her during those walks helped me to really get to know her and created some fond memories.

The key to changing your child's behavior is to do this gradually and make it fun so they do not feel they are being penalized because of their health. Start doing activities that everyone enjoys, such as playing basketball or soccer, going for walks, riding bicycles, swimming, or walking the dog. If they like the activity, they will be more inclined to leave the cell phone or TV and have some fun with you. If your child's friends are also inactive, you can either encourage all of them to join in, enroll your child in an activity without their current friends or have some one-on-one time with them.

Remember, the more fun you make exercise, the more they will want to participate. Young children are more likely to join in if you are involved. If you are not sure what activities to do, try to remember what you did when you were their age, or look on the internet as there are hundreds of resources. Remember that you cannot just tell them to be more active and then not be active yourself. They will follow your example, so if you are sitting on the couch so will they.

Physical education classes at school can play a big part in helping kids get the exercise they need, but only if these classes are offered in school and children participate. Many states in the USA do not have a statewide physical education curriculum; some schools do not have the funding to provide it while some moved money from the physical education program to fund other areas such as computer labs and library books. Schools are also accepting exemptions and waivers for these classes as students seek to avoid physical education classes due to health concerns, bullying and negative experiences.

I know that physical education class is not fun for everyone. Personally, I hated gym class because I was not an athletic person and always chosen last for every team. I was also the smallest in the class, so it didn't matter what sport we played, I got stepped on, shoved, elbowed and knocked to the ground. Dodge ball was like pinning a target on my back until I learned to hide behind the bigger kids. I understand if your child avoids gym class like the plague, but if they don't attend, then you need to ensure they get their physical activity another way.

After school babysitting can be expensive and many kids feel they are too old to be babysat but the parents want them to be active but safe. So, what is a parent to do? There are programs, such as the Boys and Girls Club in the United States or Jumpstart in Canada, that provide after school programs from age six to eighteen which promote physical activity, confidence, and community spirit. Some schools also have after school programs that children can participate in for free, and there are communities which provide free programs from 3 to 6pm during the week to help children be more active and stay safe. Check out the programs offered in your area to determine how you can safely help your child to be more active. If there are no programs available, why not contact your local politician and get them on board to create one?

Parks and playgrounds are a wonderful place for children to play and exercise, however, many parents do not allow their children to go alone because of safety concerns, distance from the home and lack of supervision. I know I never allowed my daughter to go to our local park alone as there were drug dealers and some just plain creepy guys hanging out in the park. The park was often full of empty beer cans, used needles, and other garbage. Parents are busy working, so the playgrounds sit empty while children are sitting at home in front of the television. If this is the case for you, maybe you can find someone to take your child (or a group of kids) and watch them at the park to ensure they are safe?

They say it takes a village to raise a child. Making healthy changes in the home can be difficult for low-income families, single parents, or working parents. Why not include other family members? Neighbors? Perhaps you can join together to bring about positive change for everyone.

I know of one family who had difficulty ensuring their child ate healthily or was active after school because they worked until dinner time. The parents felt there was nothing they could do until they spoke to an elderly neighbor who said she would love to have their child in her home after school. She would provide a healthy snack and play with the child and in exchange, the parents agreed to walk the neighbor's dog in the evening when it was too dark for her to leave the house. It was a win! Not only did the child get exercise before dinner, but the whole family went for a walk with the dog in the evening. I have often found once ideas get flowing, there is no end to the wonderful solutions that can be found.

Some organizations offer free passes for youth or free online programs that you can access to help ensure your child gets the exercise they need. Planet Fitness offers a *Summer Pass* for kids ages 14-19 in the United States and Canada, which includes an orientation and assistance to ensure they are lifting weights the correct way. The YMCA has a virtual ten-week program called *Generation Health* for ages 8 to 12, which provides fun activities and tracking journals to help your child move more often. There are other online resources, such as BOKS in the United States that provides games, activities and movement ideas for your child. If you can't find anything online, try contacting your local recreation center for more information or referrals.

Recipe: Taco Pasta

Ingredients
1 tsp extra virgin olive oil
5 oz (approx.) lean ground turkey or chicken
1 stalk green onion chopped
3 garlic cloves minced
1/3 tsp ground cumin
1/3 tsp chili powder
Dash of salt
1/3 large tomato diced
3 tbsp frozen corn
2 tbsp black beans cooked or from can (rinsed)
1/3 red bell pepper diced
¾ cup low sodium chicken broth
1/3 cup salsa (mild, medium or hot – you decide)
2/3 cup whole wheat pasta shells dry, uncooked

Heat oil in large skillet over medium high heat. Add the meat and break it up with a large spoon or spatula as it cooks. Once thoroughly cooked, drain excess fat.

Add onion and garlic to the pan and cook for 5 minutes.

Add cumin, chili powder, diced tomato, corn, black beans, and bell pepper. Stir and cook for 2-3 minutes.

Stir in the broth, salsa and pasta. Bring everything to boil then cover pot and reduce heat to medium-low and simmer for 15 minutes or until pasta is tender.

Remove from heat and serve immediately. Optional topping of cilantro and/or shredded cheese.

Chapter Seven: Toxins and Chemicals

"Home is where you are loved the most and act the worst."

-Marjorie Pay Hinckley

7

There is a new term being used in the scientific world called 'obesogens.' These are endocrine disrupting chemical compounds that are believed to disrupt our endocrine system, leading to an imbalance of lipid metabolism (how fats are broken down and stored in the body), metabolic issues and obesity. Obesogens are lipophilic, which means when fat is metabolized, they become free flowing therefore the body creates a fat cell to protect us.

Obesogens interfere with our metabolism and may disrupt our fat cells, so they create a greater number of fat cells (hyperplasia), or store fats more easily (hypertrophy) in the absence any changes in diet or exercise. These chemicals are found in our air, water, and every day household items such as toys, cookware, cleaning products, beauty products, lining of canned foods, and soft drink aluminum cans.

Bisphenol-A (BPA)

Most people have heard of BPA (Bisphenol-A) which is used to make polycarbonate plastics, food, and beverage containers. The problem is, it has a similar structure to estradiol (a type of the hormone estrogen) and therefore binds easily to estrogen-related receptors in the body. According to scientists, this may induce insulin resistance, inflammation in the body, oxidative stress in our cells and promote the formation of fat cells. BPA leaches from the containers into our food, drinks and beauty products and then enters the body. BPA has been banned in baby products in most countries, and in 2008, the Canadian Government listed BPA as a toxic substance and moved to force manufacturers to use alternatives. When purchasing any product, look for 'BPA Free' labels on the plastic containers.

Phthalates

Phthalates are a group of chemicals used to make plastics more flexible and durable, also often added to PVC (vinyl) products, personal care products, vinyl flooring, industrial solvents, synthetic leather, varnishes and are extremely difficult to avoid. You may see them listed as butyl benzyl phthalate (BBP), dibutyl phthalate (DBP), or di-2 ethylhexyl phthalate (DEHP). Phthalates are ingested from products that can leach into our food, inhaled from airborne particles in artificial fragrances, or absorbed through the skin from personal care products such as nail polish, hair shampoo or perfume.

In animal lab testing, DBP and DEHP damaged the reproductive system, especially on male rats. DEHP is confirmed to cause cancer in animals, but not confirmed in people. Phthalates may affect hormone receptors that are involved in metabolism, and studies have found a link between them and obesity and type 2 diabetes, but a causal link has not been established. Several studies at University of Rochester have linked phthalates to reduced rates of testosterone in men, increased belly fat, and an increased risk of fibroids.

Young children are at a greater risk because of their size, exposure to a greater number of plastic in their toys and the fact that they put everything in their mouth. Sucking and chewing can increase the risk of ingesting these chemicals. BBP, DBP and DEHP have been banned in the United States, Canada, and the European

Union, however, you may still find these chemicals in toys made in China or developing nations.

To identify if your container, toy, clothing or other product may contain phthalates, look for the number 3, 6 or 7 in the universal recycling symbol. Only microwave your food in a 'microwave safe' container. Try to use fragrance free products to avoid any phthalates that may be contained in the fragrance, especially with laundry detergent and dryer sheets as these can have a long lasting effect. Look for 'phthalate free' shampoo, cosmetics and personal care products, and use precautions when handling any cleaners or insecticides in your home that may contain these chemicals.

Atrazine

Atrazine is a common herbicide used worldwide on farms but banned in the European Union in 2004. An animal study, published in the National Library of Medicine (PMC2664469), has shown long-term exposure may decrease the basal metabolic rate, increase abdominal fat, body weight, and insulin resistance. Rats that were also fed a high fat diet, in addition to the exposure to atrazine, showed an even greater risk of obesity and insulin resistance. The Center for Disease Control (CDC) in the United States released a statement in September 2003 that stated atrazine may affect reproductive systems in humans, and caused liver, heart and kidney damage in animals. I could only find a few studies on humans and the results of these were focused primarily on pre-term birth, reproductive organs and links to cancer.

Because atrazine is commonly used with crops like corn, sweet corn, sorghum, pineapples, macadamia nuts, and sugarcane, it is best to limit your use of these products or look for organic products if you choose.

When using an herbicide in your garden that contains atrazine, be sure to wear protective gear, stay away from open windows and drinking water sources.

Perfluorooctanoic acid (PFA)

PFA (Perfluorooctanoic acid) is used in waterproof clothing, non-stick cookware, stain repellant, and microwaveable food items. The main source of human exposure is actually through contaminated water sources, and once ingested, it can remain in the body for long periods of time and has been linked to immune, thyroid, kidney, and reproductive health issues. Studies have shown an association with obesity in mice, but human studies have not been completed.

If you use non-stick cookware, use only wooden or plastic utensils in order to avoid scratching the surface. If the surface is scratched or peeling, toss it out as your family is now ingesting this product. Many microwave popcorn bags are lined with PFA, as are fast food wrappers, take out dishes, and pizza boxes. Change to air popped popcorn with unsalted butter, make your own pizza, and if you do have take-out food, transfer any leftovers to a glass container when you get home. In Canada, we can now purchase 'PFA free" products and I suspect they are available throughout the United States as well.

Synthetic Hormones

There has been a lot of controversy and discussion about hormones that are given to animals to promote faster growth and how these hormones are affecting our children. Beef are given estrogen, progesterone, and testosterone or a synthetic version of them in order to produce milk year-round or bulk up faster for slaughter. According to the Food and Drug Administration of the US, these hormones are 'safe for human consumption' but does that make them healthy? There has been some research that indicates while recombinant bovine growth hormone (rBGH) does not directly impact humans, it may increase our production of insulin-like growth factor-1 (IGF-1) which is produced in the mammary glands and the liver. High levels of IGF-1 have been associated with an increased risk of cancer of the colon, pancreas, breast, and prostate. Please note that an association with is not causation.

At this time, there is no definitive proof that hormones given to animals will cause obesity or other health issues in children. But if you are concerned, you can choose to remove beef and dairy products from your diet or look for organic hormone-free animal products.

Parabens

Parabens are chemicals that are normally used as a preservative in personal care products, such as cosmetics, shampoo, and skincare products. They are designed to kill off fungi, yeast and bacteria to improve the shelf life of a product.

Parabens may act like the hormone estrogen and can interfere with the normal production of this hormone, reproductive development, and fertility, and can increase the risk of cancer. As teenagers begin wearing makeup, deodorant, hair products, nail polish, and using skin products, their risk of exposure increases.

It is now much easier to find paraben free products in retail and drug stores across Canada, the United States and Europe. Look for 'paraben free' or read the ingredients. If it isn't listed and you aren't sure, contact the company and ask them directly.

Removing Toxins and Chemicals

I had the privilege of speaking with Lara Adler, an environmental toxin expert, and she agreed that not everyone is affected by endocrine disrupting chemicals (EDC's) the same way, but that they are linked to almost every chronic health condition. There are over 350,000 chemicals and its mixtures regulated for production, and at least 1400 are endocrine disrupting compounds. The good news is that many EDC's are non-persistent, which means we can reduce our levels by removing them from the body and avoiding further contamination.

The best way to support removal of these substances from the body is:

- To support the liver by eating highly nutritious food, especially cruciferous vegetables (broccoli, cauliflower, cabbage, kale, Bok choy and Brussell sprouts) and alliums (garlic, leeks, shallots, onions).
- Improve our air quality by opening a window, removing artificial fragrances, and scented candles.
- Purchase personal care products that are free from parabens, phthalates and BPA.
- Get a massage or exercise to improve lymphatic drainage to help remove toxins stored in the fat cells throughout the body.

Recipe: Gnocchi Pesto Salad

Ingredients:

1 tbsp extra virgin olive oil
2 cups fresh green beans
1 small package grape tomatoes
1 package (16 oz) potato gnocchi
½ cup green pesto
1 cup bite size pieces mozzarella or feta cheese

Set a large pot of water over high heat. Heat a large skillet or sauté pan over medium heat. Add the olive oil and green beans to the skillet and cook for 3 minutes, then toss in the tomatoes and continue to cook until the green beans are tender (but still crisp) and the tomatoes are browned on the outside. Then, remove from the heat.

Salt the water after it reaches a boil.

Drop the gnocchi in the boiling water and cook until they float to the surface (4 to 5 minutes).

Drain and add the gnocchi to the pan with the green beans and tomatoes. Stir in the pesto and cheese.

Divide among 4 bowls and enjoy!

Chapter Eight: Negative Influences

"Fast food chains spend a large amount of marketing to get the attention of children. People form their eating habits as children, so they try to nurture clients as youngsters.

-Eric Schlosser

8

When our children are small, we and our immediate family have the greatest impact on their dietary habits, however, as they grow, our impact is lessened by friends, school, community, the media, advertising, finances, culture, and their own personal preferences. Young children are influenced by food availability in the home (types of food and how much), eating routines (when, where and how often), what the parents are eating and their food behaviours, taste preferences, culture and age.

When your child starts school, you quickly realize you will never be able to control everything your child eats outside of the home. Children trade food, buy it from stores, or refuse to eat what you have sent for them. They want to be like their friends, which will include eating foods others do, and are popular within their community. When my daughter was in school and *one hundred calorie snack bags* became popular, all the kids at school had them. When *Lunchables* became popular, all the kids wanted them.

As a parent, it is hard to compete with your children's peers and the media, however, we can provide them healthy options and explain to them how eating these foods will make them smarter, stronger, and healthier. Make healthy natural foods appealing, serve them every day, and kids will learn to expect these foods as part of their daily diet. If the majority of their food is healthy, the occasional unhealthy option won't hurt them.

Children can be cruel, there is no doubt about it. They tease, bully, ignore, befriend, break up, and can make feeling or looking different from others the hardest thing in the world for a child. Children like to blend in and be just like everyone else around them; they want to look, talk, dress, and act just like them. Being different at school is like having a target on your back. Whether the child is special needs, taller, smaller, fatter, smarter or looks different, no child wants to stand out. So, sending an overweight child to school with a salad is just asking them to be ridiculed. But you could send a whole wheat wrap stuffed with vegetables and a delicious dip and that would be acceptable (maybe even a bit envied) or a healthy vegetable soup with pita slices or half a bagel instead of the typical sandwich on white bread. You might need to be a bit creative to convince your child to eat the healthier options at school, so talk to them and get their thoughts about changing their food at school.

Kids are going to trade food even if you tell them not to; you can ask the teacher to keep an eye on them, but let's face it, they are going to do it anyway. If you have buy-in from your child, and their food looks more appealing than those around them, they will not want to trade (at least not as much). They can declare that their lunch is better than the other person's lunch, so they do not want to trade and not be embarrassed. Work with your child to create lunches and snacks they want to eat and are okay with taking to school. There are loads of ideas on the internet for healthy lunch ideas for every age group. I like *Real Mom Nutrition*, *MOMables*, *Sarah Remmer*, and *Mums Make List*, and often recommend them to clients (I am not affiliated with them in any way), but there are many other wonderful websites you can look at for nutritious ideas. Buy them a nice water bottle to encourage them to drink water instead of juice or soft drinks.

Make sure that your child is actually eating at lunch time as pre-teens and teenagers, especially girls, will skip lunch as part of their 'diet' to try and lose weight which can promote eating disorders such as bulimia. I remember when my daughter was in grade school, a young girl would not eat her lunch because she was 'on a diet just like her mother' and would either give the food away or throw it in the garbage. This girl had a healthy weight and height and did not need to diet or restrict her calories but was influenced by what she saw at home and in the media. My daughter casually told me about it at dinner time, and the next day, I stopped at the school to speak to the principal. The school handled it beautifully by bringing in a nutritionist to talk to the whole class about why we need to eat healthy foods, how to make good choices and why it is important to eat their lunch. The young girl began to eat her lunch again and I never heard anything about it.

Sometimes kids will also say they are not hungry at dinner time, which may be because they are upset about something, severely restricting calories or perhaps because they are snacking too much after school. As a parent, you need to be aware of your child's eating habits and watch for any sudden changes. If they continue to not eat at dinner time, it is time to talk to them about it.

Because our kids spend so much time at school, working with your child's school to improve the available healthy food is imperative. Many schools no longer have vending machines full of junk food or soda. School lunch programs have improved and are providing more nutritious options. But this change did not happen magically overnight. The parents had to fight for these changes and work with the school board and principal to make these changes happen.

In my daughter's school, we fought to have the vending machines removed, and after they were gone, an enterprising young man in the fifth grade started selling chocolate bars and bags of chips out of his locker. He was eventually shut down only because he refused to give food to a kid without any money and the kid told the principal. This shows that while we removed easy access, we did not remove the cravings. Children need to be taught to want healthy foods, and removing the junk food is just the start.

If your child's school does not offer healthy options, perhaps it is time to band together with other parents and speak to your local school board. Talk to the principal about your concerns and desires. Go and speak to your Member of Parliament or Mayor. They say the 'squeaky wheel gets the oil', and I have always found that parents who work together as one voice can make amazing things happen. Insist on removing the unhealthy options, having physical education, fight for a playground and equipment to promote healthy activities and after school care that promotes physical activity in a safe environment.

There are nonprofit groups, such as the Chef Ann Foundation (CAF) that works with schools in every state across the US to provide tools, information, resources, and funding options to help create healthy food programs in schools. In Canada, the Coalition for Healthy School Food works with every province and territory to create a healthy school food program that serves culturally appropriate local food when possible. Why not look online to see what organizations exist in your area that you can work with to create healthier options for your child?

Advertising has a massive impact on our eating habits, and I would be remiss if I did not address the issue of watching television during mealtimes at home. According to a study by the University of Connecticut, fast food restaurants spent $400 million in advertising in 2012 and $5 billion dollars in 2019. With most of this advertising aimed at children, it is no wonder we have seen a huge impact on our children's health.

Watching television during mealtime is a bad idea. Not only are the commercials full of unhealthy food advertisements aimed at children, but kids also get distracted and either overeat or do not eat their meals or tell you they are finished. Then later, they will want snacks because they are hungry. According to an article in American Journal of Clinical Nutrition, when we are distracted, we eat more calories, and the more attentive we are to our meal, the less likely we are to overeat later in the same day.

Food is meant to be enjoyed and savoured, so create a habit of eating together as a family without the distractions of television, computers or cellphone. Ban cellphones from the table (including the adults) and talk about your day, current events, activities coming up or better yet, ask them about theirs. Getting your children talking is a wonderful thing as it makes them feel wanted, important and that their opinion matters. Eating together as a family also slows down the speed of eating, which allows the body to realize it is full and send the leptin hormone to the brain to signal us to stop eating.

Food manufacturers spend millions of dollars advertising to children. If you watch the type of commercials that are shown during after school hours, you will see sugary cereal, snack bars, ice cream, instant foods, fast food restaurants, soda and more. The advertisers know that children are greatly affected by their colourful advertisements and will start asking the parents to purchase these foods. Vitamin water is a perfect example; it is water with flavouring and sweeteners, has no added health benefits and is completely unnecessary, but the advertising for this product has made it hugely popular with teenagers. By limiting the time your children are influenced by the media, you will be improving their physical and emotional health and saving yourself money in the process.

Media not only negatively affects our children by promoting unhealthy foods, but body types as well. As I spoke about earlier, we are bombarded by advertisements for cosmetics, skin care, clothing and most show a young thin woman with flawless skin who is under weight. Young girls have enough pressure on them without having to live up to unrealistic expectations. Talk to your child about what a healthy weight means and how they should focus on being strong, active and happy with themselves and not worry about looking like an air brushed underweight model in a magazine.

There is a great video on *Huff Post* that demonstrates the air brushing and alterations that advertisers use, and I strongly encourage you to show this to your daughter. You can find it on YouTube under https://youtu.be/17j5QzF3kqE and the video shows how unrealistic these models are. In the last few years, advertisers have started showing models in a variety of sizes and body types, but I find the majority of them are still unrealistic.

Recipe: Lunch Wrap

Wraps are a great alternative to the traditional sandwich because they have less sugar than bread and you can fill them with delicious vegetables.

Ingredients

1 whole wheat or spinach wrap
Mustard or pesto sauce
Bell peppers sliced
Onions sliced
2 pieces lettuce or kale
3 slices cucumber
¼ cup black beans cooked or from can
¼ cup shredded carrots
¼ cup cooked brown rice or quinoa
¼ cup cooked meat (chicken, pork or tuna)

Spread the sauce on the wrap, then layer toppings in the middle. Tuck in both ends and roll together. Wrap in wax paper to keep from breaking apart (also serves as a placemat to catch the extras).

Tip:

Avoid too much sauce as it will make the wrap soggy by lunchtime.

If serving immediately, include slices of avocado.

Serve with napkins.

Chapter Nine: Our Relationship with Food

"Being healthy isn't about inches, pounds or how kids look – it's about how they feel and making sure they feel good about themselves. So, rather than focusing on appearance, it's important to emphasize to kids that when we eat healthy food and stay active, we feel better, and can perform better in everything we do, from athletics to academics."

-Michelle Obama

9

Think of every social event you have ever been to, and food is a main part of the event: sweet birthday cake with candles, tiered wedding cake, summer barbeques with burgers, beer and chips, celebrations for anniversaries at restaurants, and even dating all feature food. While I am writing this chapter, I am planning out a birthday party for my husband and creating a menu for our guests. While I want the food to be healthy, I know there is an expectation to provide popular snack foods that are less than healthy, as well as a birthday cake.

From ancient to modern times, the events in our lives are marked with food. It connects us with other people, provides good feelings, comfort, reinforces cultural traditions and gives us a feeling of community. Eating together also helps our mental health and avoid feelings of isolation, depression and loneliness.

Food is far more than just nutrition and has become part of our cultural norms. Culture affects our body weight and perceptions of what is normal, and from the time we are little, we look to our parents and extended family to learn what is normal behaviour. If the parents are physically active or play sports, then chances are that the children will as well. If the parents are overweight, the children will usually be as well. A part of it is genetics, but a large part is learned behaviour. We are also influenced by our peers and the body shape that is promoted by society at the time.

Back in the 1940s, the voluptuous sweater girl with large perky breasts was the style. Then in the 1960s, being thin like the model Twiggy was all the rage. In the

1980s, being athletic was the desired shape, and in the 1990s, it changed to being extremely thin with protruding collar bones and ankles. In 2010, a large booty became popular with the celebrities taking it to the extreme.

Throughout history, the cultural desired look has changed from extremely thin to being overweight. In some cultures, gaining weight is desired, and children of normal weight are 'too skinny.' Being overweight may be associated with strength, wealth, and fertility, and if other members of the family are overweight or obese, the child is more likely to gain weight to fit into the family dynamic.

Children of overweight parents are more likely to be overweight due to diet, exercise habits, genetics and also because they want to fit in and be just like their parents. If you ever talk to a child that is different from the rest of their family, one of the common complaints is how they feel like an outsider. If the family members are of average weight and very athletic and one person is overweight – that person will feel out of place. If the members of the family and/or community are overweight, the healthy weight child will change their habits to gain weight to fit in with their family.

Time for some tough love. If you are overweight, part of healing your child will be healing yourself. Just as you love your child no matter their size, you need to love yourself the same way. Focus on making changes for the entire family to be healthier, not just on losing weight. While this book was written for children and teenagers, the nutrition information applies to adults as well. Your child is looking to you for guidance and will model your behaviour. If you want a healthy happy child, you need to adopt a healthy lifestyle as well.

Along with trying to fit in, kids may also be dealing with that well-meaning friend or relative that is always pushing food or encouraging them to eat more; perhaps a grandparent or aunt who will not let them leave their house without eating something. Food pushers are a real thing, and dealing with them can be a bit tricky. On one hand, you do not want to upset your well-meaning friend or family member, but on the other hand, you have the health and well-being of your child to consider.

Here are a few tips that might help you.

- Do not visit during mealtimes (this usually gets you out of several helpings of a meal) but not out of snacks or drinks.
- Tell them you just ate (be warned, they will tell you it is not as good as theirs so you need more, and will want to give you food), and if they push food on you, tell them you would love to take it home to eat it later. Then ask for a glass of water so you are accepting something from them, because food pushers need to give you something.
- Explain that your doctor has advised your child needs to follow a specific diet. Truthfully, this one is a bit harder because they will argue their food is healthy, and they know better than the doctor. It can also make the child feel extremely uncomfortable.
- Explain low glycemic eating and how it affects blood sugar levels, so the family is now only eating certain foods. Honestly, trying to convince someone else that their eating habits

are unhealthy is exceedingly difficult without insulting them. For children, this can be impossible, and they end up feeling pressured to conform.

If your child is only attending a few celebratory occasions a year, such as birthdays or Christmas dinner, I suggest you enjoy the celebration and not worry about what they are eating. However, if celebrations occur more regularly, then you may need to decide on a way to ensure they are eating healthier. Options could be eating a healthy snack before they go to the event, which will help keep them from eating as much unhealthy foods. Or offer to send food with your child to help the host and ensure the food is something healthy they can eat (this works well with children with allergies or diabetes).

Discuss with your child whatever strategy they feel comfortable with, which will depend on their age and buy-in with the healthier lifestyle. Unless they have a health issue (such as diabetes), they can enjoy a piece of cake at a birthday party without any effects and denying them may cause more harm than good.

Another issue that is now affecting children and teenagers is being overweight or obese is becoming 'normal', and some children are gaining weight to fit in with what their peers expect. We have all heard the expression, 'you are the average of the five people you associate with most', which means if the people you spend time together with are active, fit, and energetic, then you are more likely to conform. If the people you associate with are overweight, sedentary and care less about their diet, then you will do the same. As more children and teenagers gain weight, they become less active and have poor diets, same as their peers.

Motivating change in children and teenagers may also require dealing with their peers, extended family members and teachers. You may need to include their friends in healthier activities in order to have more support from your child. The more buy-in you create to change your diet and lifestyle, the easier and more effective it will be. Never yell, bribe, punish, or threaten your child about their weight, food, or exercise. If these issues turn into fights, the results can be harmful. The more kids feel worse about their weight, the more likely they are to binge eat or develop an eating disorder.

Remember, food is nutrition and should never be used as a punishment or reward. Do not send them to bed without dinner if they misbehave or promise a sweet treat for a good report card. Alternatively, do not use food as a reward for exercise. You cannot out exercise a bad diet, and this can cause eating disorders down the road. It is important to know that food is only for nutrition, not for comfort, reward, or punishment. Compliment them when they choose a healthier option, such as playing basketball outside rather than sitting and watching television, but do not focus on weight loss. Let this change be all about being healthier and more active as a family.

When you are out in public, especially around peers or family, there will be times when you see what food or how much food your child is eating, and you are going to have to bite your tongue and not say anything. Seriously, kids do not respond to nagging or shaming, especially in front of their peers or strangers. Wait until the right time and a private place to have these conversations, about food portions or what types of food to eat, in a safe and non-judgmental way.

Food can also be a source of comfort for children, especially those who are feeling lonely, scared, or anxious. Food we enjoy creates dopamine (that feel good hormone), which encourages us to eat more of it. We can use food to fill a void in our emotional health because it makes us feel good (at least for the moment) or remind us of a previous occasion when we felt happy. During times of stress, such as when parents are fighting, or a parent is ill, or difficulties at school; children may use food as a coping mechanism for their stress. Talk to your child about how they are feeling and encourage them to use other methods to address the emotions they are feeling, such as colouring, drawing, journaling, exercise, or other coping methods.

As a parent, you are the biggest influence on your child's eating habits, and you will need to change your relationship with food to model healthy eating habits for your child. When you are bored, stressed, sad or anxious – do you turn to food? What other behaviours can you adopt rather than turning to food?

Our kids watch what we do, and they repeat our patterns of behaviour. So, if you want to help your child, you need to help yourself. I never realized how my daughter was watching my behaviour until the day I was really stressed out and she made a comment about buying the McCain cake. When she is stressed out, she also turns to food for comfort and now both of us are working on changing our habits.

Recipe: Grilled Pineapple and Chicken Salad

Ingredients:

2 tbsp extra virgin olive oil
1 ½ tsp apple cider vinegar
1 ½ tsp maple syrup
8 oz chicken breast
1 ½ cups pineapple cut into rings
3 cups baby spinach
½ cup blueberries
½ avocado diced
¼ cup feta cheese crumbled
¼ cup red onion thinly sliced

Add 1 tbsp olive oil, apple cider vinegar, maple syrup, to a small mason jar. Shake and set aside.

Preheat grill on medium heat. Brush both sides of chicken breast with remaining olive oil. Cook 15 to 20 minutes flipping halfway until cooked thoroughly. Cook pineapple until grill marks appear, about six minutes each side.

Meanwhile, toss together spinach, blueberries, feta, avocado and red onion in a large bowl. Chop pineapple into chunks and chicken into strips or chunks. Add to salad. Serve on individual plates and top with dressing.

Chapter Ten: Cravings and Habits

"People do not decide their futures, they decide their habits and their habits decide their futures."

-F. Matthias Alexander

10

Cravings can occur because of habit, hunger, or emotions. As humans, we like our habits because it makes life easier, but if we have an unhealthy habit, it can be difficult to break. Maybe your child has ice cream for dessert every night? Or do they crave sugary foods in the afternoon? Or do they ask for food from McDonald's restaurant every time you are out? All of these are habits, but the reasons for the habits may be different. Children develop habits the same way we do, and it is important to understand and recognize their current habits in order to create healthier ones.

Notice whether they are craving food because they are bored, stressed, out of habit, or actually hungry; then you will be able to distract them, talk to them or give them a healthy snack. Ensuring your child eats a filling breakfast, doesn't skip meals, and has protein, healthy fat, and carbohydrates with each meal, can go a long way in preventing the afternoon sugar craving or snacking after dinner.

Kids can get into eating habits very quickly. My granddaughter is only two years old, and she can recognize the McDonald's sign when we are out and will start asking for fries. If you know you are going to a place where they will be tempted and start asking for food, then bring a healthy snack with you to offer them, or (depending on the age) you can just tell them 'no, we will eat when we get home.' If you give in to their demand every time, you are reinforcing a bad habit, but if you don't, you are training their healthy eating habits for the future.

If your daughter has pre-menstrual cravings caused by the change in progesterone and estrogen, providing a complex carbohydrate (such as beans, lentils, brown rice) and sweet tasting berries can go a long way to help prevent the cravings for carbs and sugar. Chocolate cravings have been linked to a low level of magnesium, so dark leafy greens, seeds and whole grains can help address these cravings. If she is craving salty foods, this usually means she is dehydrated, and the body may be trying to manage her sodium levels. A green smoothie, cold green tea or plain water may help rehydrate her and make those salt cravings disappear.

When a craving hits, I know it can be hard to fight. You can try and distract yourself with an activity, have a glass of water or exercise. Many dieticians will tell you to find a healthier option that will fulfill the craving (such as having strawberries when you are craving something sweet), but in my practice, I have found that this really does not work. I found that clients eat multiple foods to try and fulfill the craving (eating a huge number of calories), yet the craving is still there. But if they just eat a small amount of that specific food, the craving would be satisfied, and fewer calories consumed.

Another way to stop a craving is to have the opposite taste. For example, if you crave something sweet, eat something sour and the craving will disappear. Sounds weird, right? By eating something sour, you are stimulating your taste buds which will distract you from the craving. This is why people who want to quit smoking finds brushing their teeth with mint toothpaste will often stop cigarette cravings.

A healthy life is about balance, and just because your family is now eating healthy does not mean that your child cannot have their favourite treat food now and again. I love cake and pie and I could eat it every day (I have a serious sweet tooth), but I don't because I know it is not a healthy option. I allow myself to have a piece of cake or pie once a month on my free day, and just knowing I can have it usually gets rid of any cravings I have. Life is not all or nothing, and as long as your child is not medically restricted from a food or food group, having some balance in their diet will be easier and emotionally healthier.

Recipe: Slow Cooker Pork with Vegetables

Ingredients:

1 Pork Loin or roast
2 potatoes (peeled and cubed)
4 carrots (peeled and sliced)
½ onion (diced)
Montreal steak spice or any of your seasoning of choice
1 head broccoli

In the morning, place pork in slow cooker and season with spices. Then, place potatoes, carrots and onion on top. Add ¼ cup water. Cover and turn on low and cook until suppertime.

Steam broccoli over the stove or in microwave.

Cut up meat and serve with vegetables on individual plates.

Tip:

You can change the broccoli for green beans, cauliflower or a side salad.

Use the leftover meat in a soup or wraps for lunch tomorrow.

Chapter Eleven: The Impact of Stress

"In your most challenging parenting moments, take a deep breath and try to remember that the moment your child is at their most challenging is the moment your child is struggling with the most challenges."

-Unknown

11

When we are feeling stress, anxiety, worry or fear, our body releases cortisol (the stress hormone) which creates a release of glucose (sugars) in the blood stream for immediate energy in case we need to run away. Cortisol narrows the arteries, while another hormone called epinephrine increases your heart rate. This allows the body to pump the blood faster, allowing you to deal with the immediate threat. Now, this is fine for short term events like when you are late and running for the bus or away from an angry dog, but what if this reaction is chronic?

Because cortisol releases glucose in the body through a process called gluconeogenesis to provide immediate energy, chronic cortisol creates persistent high sugar levels in the blood (called hyperglycemia). With this constant demand, the pancreas may struggle to keep up, and if unable to do so, diabetes will occur.

Without sufficient insulin, cells are starved for nutrients and can cause the brain to release ghrelin, the hormone that tells us we are hungry and need to eat, even if we do not need more food. False food signals lead to overeating and weight gain.

Cortisol also suppresses the immune system, making us susceptible to cold, flu and disease. Digestion is also shut down as it is not needed during times of imminent threat, and chronic stress can create digestive issues such as irritable bowel syndrome, heart burn, and lack of nutrition absorption.

Chronic narrowing of the arteries and high blood pressure can lead to blood vessel damage, causing heart disease and plaque build up in the arteries. While the heart is designed to help us move, especially during times of danger, chronic stress, anxiety, and fear can damage the heart over time. Stress can create havoc with the body and disrupt their normal sleep and growth patterns, creating weight gain, hormonal imbalance, and mental health issues.

As adults, we rarely think about a child feeling stressed out, after all, they are not responsible for going to work and paying the bills, so what do they have to be stressed about? Stress can come from a variety of sources, and not just events or people. According to an article in the Journal of Caring Sciences, approximately thirty five percent of children experience stress related health problems that require a physician's care.

In my day, if you did something stupid, it would be over in a day or so (or when I stopped being grounded by my parents). Now, these events are caught on cellphone cameras and live on forever online on social media. When I was a child, the newspaper came once a day during the week, and since I did not read the newspaper, I was happily oblivious to the negative events in the world. Now, kids have instant messaging on their cellphones that tells them of news stories around the world. If there is a shooting at a school in another state, they see horrible images, video interviews and can replay the event over and over, creating fear and stress. They have school shooting drills that can create a traumatic event reaction even if it was not real.

Kids can be bullied or pressured online from hundreds of 'friends' and even children as young as six years old have reported issues from social media pressure. They now see more images of violence in video games and on television than ever before. According to a study published by Harvard University, "exposure to violence is associated with elevated risk for a wide range of mental health problems in children and adolescents, including depression, anxiety and post-traumatic stress disorder."

Another cause of stress can be trying to be 'perfect;' Wear the perfect outfit, have the perfect hair style, be the perfect size, and be the perfect student or friend. Trying to be perfect is exhausting and stressful but can manifest as a form of control of their environment. When I was a teenager, I was one of those kids. My room was perfectly clean, hair was perfect, grades had to be A's, or I would feel out of control and unworthy. It was a form of stress manifestation, but a wise woman told me 'a beautiful thing is never perfect', and she talked to me about what was causing my stress and ways to deal with it. I was lucky she was there, but many young people are doing their best to deal with massive stress without any help from others.

Here are a few examples of causes of stress that your child may be exposed to:
- Being alone at home for long periods of time can create fear and loneliness.
- Social Media, cameras everywhere, and having life out there for everyone to see and judge.
- Bullying or peer pressure – in person and online.
- Trying to fit in.
- Pleasing family members or being the peace maker in the family.

- Worrying about grades, exams, or homework.
- Online schooling.
- Experiencing discrimination or hate.
- Tensions at home can create chronic stress, especially if parents are divorcing.
- Puberty and hormone changes.
- World events, school shootings, violence in hometown, can create traumatic stress as children may be exposed in real life or through the media.
- Violence on television, movies, and video games can create a stress response in the body.
- Fewer physical outlets for stress.
- Lack of sleep.
- Poor diet.
- Chronic illness such as asthma, ADHD, obesity and learning disabilities.

Children may not be able to understand nor express that they are feeling stress, and as parents, we will see other behaviours instead. Depending on their age, you will see different indicators such as:

- Tantrums.
- Whining.
- Clinging or not wanting to be apart from a parent.
- Withdraw from or not want to interact with friends or family.
- Nightmares or trouble sleeping or excessive sleeping.
- Stomach or headaches.
- Difficulty concentrating.

- Change in eating habits such as not eating or excessive eating.
- Negative self talk.
- Breaking curfew and acting out or cutting class.
- Trying to be perfect and extreme controlling of their environment.

As I've explained, stress can have a negative impact on your child's weight and wellbeing. If you believe your child is suffering from stress or anxiety, it is important to talk to them and not dismiss their feelings. We may think of the issue as insignificant, but to the child, these feelings are big and a real problem they cannot resolve on their own. If you are not successful in helping your child talk through an issue, please consider getting them professional help. School counsellors, church ministers, or a mental health professional are there to help you and your family. There are also children's help lines they can call for free help if they need it.

Recipe: Salmon with Green Beans

Ingredients:

2 cups green beans (washed and trimmed)
1 cup cherry tomatoes
1 ½ tsp extra virgin olive oil
Salt and pepper to taste
10 oz salmon fillet

Preheat oven to 510 degrees.

Place beans and tomatoes in a bowl and toss with the olive oil. Season with salt and pepper. Transfer to a nonstick baking sheet or lined with parchment paper and bake in oven for 10 minutes.

Season salmon fillets with pepper.

Remove vegetables from oven and place salmon fillets over top. Place back in the oven and bake 7 to 10 minutes or until salmon flakes with a fork.

Divide vegetables between plates and top with salmon.

Tip:

Serve with quinoa or brown rice for a more filling meal.

Chapter Twelve: Unexplained Weight Gain

"Behind weight gain are the larger hurts and questions
that have to be explored, probed and understood before
weight loss and maintenance is a possibility. It's a
bigger issue than just calories in and calories out."

-Ali Vincent

12

It is common for teenagers to suddenly gain weight because of puberty, more freedom of food choices, growth spurts or changes in body shape (some fill out then grow taller). There are also rare occasions where a teenager will have unexplained weight gain that cannot be attributed to excess calories, a poor diet, or a lack of exercise. Some of these situations are a misfunctioning pituitary gland, a tumour on the pituitary gland, Polycystic Ovary Syndrome, thyroid imbalance, or hormonal imbalance. Each of these situations will be assessed and diagnosed by a doctor.

The pituitary gland is a pea sized gland located at the base of the brain that controls growth, metabolism, and hormone production. Pituitary tumours cause a condition called Cushing Disease, which is normally associated with fatty deposits on the upper back and stomach area, rounded face and pink or purple stretch marks on the skin. People with Cushing Disease bruise easily, feel weak and tired and often have high blood pressure. Your doctor will do a variety of saliva, urine, and blood tests to measure levels of cortisol and determine the best course of action.

Polycystic Ovary Syndrome (PCOS) is associated with high levels of androgens (male hormones) in women of childbearing age. They often have irregular menstrual cycles, cysts on the ovaries (but not all women with PCOS have cysts), excess hair on face, back or buttocks, a loss of hair on the head, weight gain and difficulty getting pregnant. There is no cure for PCOS, but a diet low in simple carbohydrates and inflammatory foods has been shown to alleviate some of the symptoms. In my book *PCOS: Symptom Solutions*, I include a menu plan that removes inflammatory foods such as sugar, dairy, and processed meats, provide information on supplements that may help and offer advice on exercise programs. I have found that some doctors will not diagnose PCOS unless the women have at least four of the symptoms, while other doctors are not as rigid. If you suspect your daughter has PCOS, I recommend seeing an endocrinologist who will be able to diagnose and assist you.

The thyroid gland is located in the neck and is shaped like a butterfly. Low functioning thyroid must be assessed by your physician through a blood test. When checking your thyroid, the doctor will check their T3, T4 and thyroid antibodies and will prescribe thyroid medication if required. Selenium is a mineral required in the body in a very small quantity but is needed to convert T4 to T3. Some natural sources of selenium are Brazil nuts, walnuts, mushrooms, fish, avocados and some cereal grains, and including these in your diet can support the thyroid gland.

Hormonal imbalances are rare in children but will also be assessed with a series of blood tests. Symptoms include growth failure, muscle weakness, fatigue, easy bruising, obesity, high blood pressure, depression and anxiety. If your doctor suspects a hormonal imbalance, you should be referred to an endocrinologist.

Recipe: Cauliflower Fried Rice

Ingredients:

1 head of cauliflower florets
2 tbsp extra virgin olive oil
2 eggs (beaten) *optional
2 cloves garlic (minced)
¾ cup carrots (peeled and diced into pea size)
¾ cup peas (fresh or frozen and defrosted)
½ cup white or red onion (diced)
2 tbsp low sodium soy sauce
2 tbsp green onions (diced)

Heat medium size skillet over medium-high heat. Once hot add 1 tbsp oil, garlic and cook for 30 seconds. Add carrots and cook for 2 minutes until tender.

Add peas and cook for 1 minute.

Add cauliflower and stir to combine. Spread out evenly in the pan to cook without stirring, about 2 minutes.

Mix and continue frying until tender. About 5 minutes. Add soy sauce, stirring to combine.

*Make a well in the middle of the mixture. Add 1 tbsp oil to center. Once hot, add in eggs and stir quickly to scramble. Once cooked, stir all ingredients again.

Garnish with green onion and serve.

Part B: The Solutions

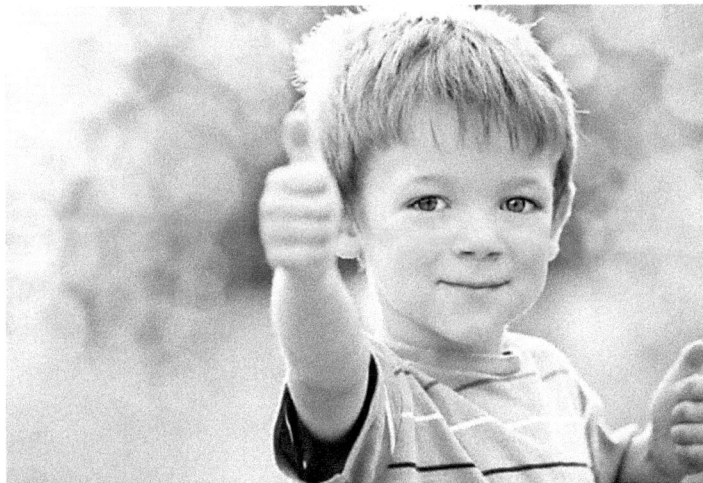

Chapter Thirteen: How Our Body Works

"Today, more than 95% of all chronic disease is caused by food choice, toxic food ingredients, nutritional deficiencies and lack of physical exercise."

-Mike Adams

13

I know I told you that this book would not be filled with complicated medical terminology, but I believe it is important for you to understand how the body works. Knowledge is power, and knowledge about the body can help you create a healthy diet for your family. Let's look at a simple explanation of how our body is designed, for clues on how we are supposed to be eating.

Our body consists of trillions of cells that work as a whole to support homeostasis (staying constant), which ensures our internal environment is safe and healthy. Each body system contributes to this homeostasis in a specific way. For example, the level of glucose – a building block of fruits, vegetables, and sweets - is maintained in our blood stream. Our body does this because glucose is a source of energy for our cells. For example, the brain needs a steady supply of glucose, or energy, to stay functioning and low levels of glucose may lead to unconsciousness, coma or even death. Our body regulates the amount of glucose in the blood with the use of insulin produced by the pancreas. If we ingest too much glucose, it will be stored for future use in our liver, our muscles and in the form of fat cells. When there isn't enough glucose in the blood stream, the brain triggers our body to release the glucose we have stored to keep our brain and body working efficiently. It is this cycle that prompts the body to trigger hunger; to replace whatever vitamins, nutrients, glucose, and other minerals that were used up by the body throughout the day.

The process of eating and preparing food for our cells is broken down into six basic functions: ingestion, secretion, mixing and propulsion, digestion, absorption, and defecation. In this way, the healthy body can be like a well-oiled machine that runs smoothly and efficiently. It takes in larger food items and then breaks it down into the molecules like glucose that our body needs to stay healthy.

In our stomach, the muscles use our digestive juices to mix the food and the liquids we ingested, in order to break it into smaller pieces. Fats are broken into fatty acids, proteins into amino acids, and carbohydrates into glucose, galactose and fructose which are eventually converted to glucose. This mixture (called chyme) is slowly moved into our small intestine where the walls of the small intestine absorb the water and digest nutrients into our blood stream through tiny, hair-like projections called villi. From the small intestine, leftover undigested food and some water is moved into the large intestine. In the large intestine, healthy bacteria break down the proteins and starches that were not broken down in the small intestine. The large intestine absorbs water and insoluble fibre sticks to the remaining products that are ready to form into stool. Insoluble fibre speeds up the movement of this waste product and prevents constipation and blockage. I will explain the importance of fibre later in this chapter. Once formed into stool, it is moved to the rectum to be removed via the anus during a bowel movement.

Fats

Fats have building blocks called fatty acids, which are broken down into three categories based on the number of hydrogen atoms that make them up. *Saturated fats* are found primarily in animal products and are normally solid at room temperature. You see this type of fat in the marbling in animal meat, cheese, and butter. Coconut oil and palm kernel oil are also high in saturated fats. Our liver uses these fats to create cholesterol and excessive dietary intake can raise the blood cholesterol levels (especially the low-density lipoproteins or 'bad' cholesterol), which are a major factor in high blood pressure, obesity, heart disease, stroke and colon cancer.

Polyunsaturated fats are found in corn, safflower, soybean and sunflower oils as well as some fish oils. These oils may lower our high-density lipoproteins or 'good cholesterol,' are high in calories and should be kept to a minimum in the diet. These vegetable oils are found in most highly processed foods. The exception are the *omega-3 fatty acids* found in cold water fish and flaxseed oil, which do not affect our cholesterol levels and help to reduce the risk of heart disease. We should try to increase our omega-3 fats and reduce our intake of the above vegetable oils, especially in processed foods.

Monounsaturated fats are found mostly in vegetable and nut oils such as canola, peanut and olive oil. Research suggests that they reduce our bad LDL cholesterol but do not impact our good HDL cholesterol. I personally do not use canola oil because of the way it is processed, nor do I use peanut oil because of allergies. When I use oil in our salad dressings or for stir fried vegetables, I use cold pressed extra virgin olive oil.

You should be aware that most plant oils contain a mixture of the three types of fatty acids, but we categorize it based on what it is mostly comprised of. We need fat in our diet because it can be broken down into glucose for energy, absorb fat-soluble vitamins (A, D, E and K), form cell membranes and help to regulate hormones. Healthy fats contribute to soft smooth hair and skin, bright eyes, and healthy joints.

Carbohydrates

Carbohydrates supply our body with energy and are only found mostly in plants (fruits, vegetables, grains) and milk products. They are classified as either *simple carbohydrates,* or *complex carbohydrates. Simple carbohydrates* include fructose (from fruit), sucrose (refined sugar) or lactose (milk sugar). *Complex carbohydrates* are made up of sugar molecules that are strung together to form longer more complex chains and include fibre, starches and vegetables. Both types are converted into glucose to be used by the body. Carbohydrates are the body's main source of glucose, which is used as fuel for the cells and the only source of fuel for the brain and red blood cells.

Protein

Protein is needed for growth and development, manufacturing hormones, antibodies, enzymes and tissues. When we consume protein, it is broken down into amino acids. Amino acids may be created by both animal and plant sources and are classified into three types:
1. Essential
2. Nonessential
3. Conditionally essential

Since our body cannot produce essential amino acids, we must ingest them from our food. The nine essential amino acids are: histidine, isoleucine, leucine, lysine, methionine, phenylalanine, threonine, tryptophan and valine. Common food sources that contain essential amino acids are beef, poultry, fish, eggs, soy, dairy, quinoa, and buckwheat.

Nonessential amino acids can be produced by our body even if we don't eat the right foods. These amino acids include asparagine, aspartic acid, alanine, cysteine, glutamine, glycine, proline, serine, and tyrosine.

Conditionally essential amino acids are normally made in the body but may be essential depending on our diet, illness and stress. These amino acids include arginine, cysteine, glutamine, tyrosine, glycine, proline and serine. Eating a balanced healthy diet with complete proteins ensures we have the building blocks for all the amino acids we require.

There are two types of proteins, depending on which amino acids they provide – complete and incomplete. *Complete proteins* contain all the essential amino acids and are found in meat, fish, poultry, cheese, eggs and milk. *Incomplete proteins* contain only some of the essential amino acids and are found in grains, legumes and leafy vegetables.

To make a complete protein, complementary incomplete protein sources are combined. This means that we plan to eat certain foods that are lacking a particular amino acid with another food that has that specific amino acid. It is not necessary to eat both at the same time as research shows our body can store these throughout the day. Examples of complementary proteins are beans with:
1.   Brown rice

2.   Corn
3.   Nuts
4.   Seeds
5.   Wheat

Or combine brown rice with:
1.   Beans
2.   Nuts
3.   Seeds

The daily protein requirements for children are dependent on their age, height and weight. When they are teenagers, their activity and muscle mass starts to play a role as well. The following amounts are approximate minimum total daily protein requirements.
1.   Babies 10 grams
2.   School aged kids 19-34 grams
3.   Teenage boys up to 52 grams
4.   Teenage girls 46 grams

Kids require 1 to 1.5grams of protein for every TWO pounds of weight, or 1 gram per kilogram of weight. For example, a 32 lb (14.51 kg) toddler would require 14 grams of protein, which isn't very much.

For example:
1.   1 large egg (6 grams)
2.   8oz milk (8 grams)
3.   1 cup cooked oatmeal (6 grams)
4.   1 cup green peas (9 grams)
5.   4 oz lean beef (28 grams)
6.   2 oz turkey breast (16 grams)
7.   1 medium baked potato (5 grams)

As parents, we wonder if we are giving enough protein to our children, but according to an article in the National

Health and Nutrition Examination survey (Nils-Gerrit Wunsch, Nov 30, 2021) the average intake of protein was higher than required, especially from animal sources. They indicated that males aged two to five were consuming 56.7 grams, aged six to eleven were consuming 68.8 grams, and twelve to nineteen years were consuming 86.5 grams. There is such a thing as too much protein intake.

Symptoms of excessive protein include:
- Weight gain (due to excess calories).
- Kidney stones.
- High levels of nitrogen in the liver (makes liver work harder to process out waste and toxins).
- Bad breath.
- Constipation.
- Heart disease.

To give you a real-life example, I asked a friend of mine what animal protein her ten-year-old son ate last Saturday, and she told me he ate four slices of bacon, one egg, a big mac, a glass of milk, and six chicken nuggets. This is 123 grams of protein and almost 2500 calories! While the human body can handle a lot of protein, it is important to understand that 'protein' isn't stored in the body, but the excess is converted to glucose and stored as fat.

Regardless of whether we eat more carbohydrates, fats or proteins, the excess is stored in our fat cells (adipose tissue) as glucose to be used later for energy. There is some debate in the scientific community whether we are born with a specific number of fat cells that enlarge as we store excess calories, or whether we create more fat cells, but regardless, if we consume more than required it is stored as fat.

Plants, whole grains and animal products have plenty of protein for your growing child, and if you are feeding your child a well-balanced diet with a variety of food, then they are probably getting enough. I tell my clients to aim for one third of the meal as animal protein (dairy, fish, poultry, beef, pork, eggs) and the other two thirds as plant-based foods. If you want to track your child's meals to ensure you are serving enough protein, you can use online free apps, which will also tell you their vitamin and mineral intake or *My Health Tracker for Kids* available on Amazon, which I created to work in conjunction with this book.

Water

Water is essential to life and is involved in every function in our body. It helps to transport nutrients to our cells and waste from the cell out of the body. We need it for digestion, absorption, absorbing water-soluble vitamins, excretion of waste products and maintaining our body temperature. Each day we lose water through breathing, urine, perspiration, and feces; a total of approximately six to ten cups. We need to replace this fluid either by drinking water or through eating fruits and vegetables that contain water. You can tell whether you are dehydrated by the colour of your urine. If it is a pale yellow, you are properly hydrated. Dark yellow to orange (usually with a strong smell) means you are dehydrated.

Fibre

Fibre performs a crucial role in our digestive system and there are two types of fiber in our diet, both of which are necessary for optimal health. *Soluble fiber* from nuts, seeds, beans, oat bran and some fruits and vegetables break down in water and form a gel-like material, slowing digestion (which keeps you feeling full longer). This type of fiber is also prebiotic, meaning they feed the good bacteria in our gut that promote a healthy immune system. *Soluble fibre* also absorbs excess fat, helping lower cholesterol and blood sugar levels.

Insoluble fiber does not break down in fluids but absorbs them and sticks to other materials, which adds bulk to our stool. This allows waste to pass more easily from the body. *Insoluble fiber* prevents constipation, improves bowel health, and aids in removing waste products from the body. Some sources of *insoluble fiber* include brown rice, whole grains, couscous, carrots, parsnips, beans, lentils, peas, nuts and seeds. You may have noticed that some of the foods that contain *insoluble fiber* also contain *soluble fiber.*

We need natural sources of fiber every day and since many plants contain both types of fiber, it is easy to incorporate these helpful foods into our diet. Children that eat a diet of highly processed foods, meat, dairy and insufficient water do not consume enough fiber, which can cause constipation, pain, diverticulitis, hemorrhoids, inflammation in the bowels and ultimately colon cancer.

Artificial fiber sources, such as a fiber supplement, do not provide the same benefit to the body as they are not prebiotic, and they do not provide the same vitamins, minerals, and nutrients as natural foods. We need to ingest prebiotic foods to feed our gut bacteria and maintain a healthy immune system.

Over seventy percent of a healthy immune system is built in the gut, and to have a healthy gut, we need to feed the one hundred trillion good bacteria living there and remove the foods and toxins that are harming our gut. These microorganisms help control our digestion, communicate with our brain, control hormone production, and produce nutrients such as Vitamin K. Eating foods that are good prebiotics, such as artichokes, mushrooms, bananas, cabbage, asparagus, red kidney beans and chickpeas, helps to ensure the health of our gut and immunity.

Fermented foods contain probiotics that contribute to our microbiome but not all fermented foods contain live probiotics. Naturally fermented foods such as yogurt, kefir, kimchi, and sauerkraut will contain the helpful probiotics if they have the words 'naturally fermented' or 'contains live cultures' on the label. Sadly, pasteurization and preservatives kill beneficial bacteria, which means if you are buying flavoured sweetened yogurt thinking it contains probiotics – it might not. You can usually tell naturally fermented foods because they have a slight sour or tangy taste.

Immunity

Our health is dependent upon absorbing nutrients in the small intestine via villi and microvilli: hair-like extensions along the inside of small intestine. Healthy natural food contributes vitamins, minerals, phytonutrients and fiber to our body while a diet of highly processed foods, high sugar foods, and artificial ingredients causes inflammation and disease.

Because a lack of nutrients impacts our immune system; children who lack correct nutrition are more prone to illness, disease, and chronic long term health issues. Scientific studies have demonstrated that children with behavioural issues, anxiety and depression often lack specific nutrients, and when these nutrients are added back into the diet, the issues are alleviated, or disappear. While there is no conclusive data showing a lack of nutrients causes Attention Deficit Hyperactivity Disorder (ADHD), it has been shown that seventy-eight percent of children diagnosed with ADHD have nutrient deficiencies.

Other symptoms we may see in a child that is lacking nutrients include: canker sores inside the mouth, dry hair or skin, brittle nails, bleeding gums, difficulty seeing in low light, fatigue, constant colds, and flu.

When we need energy, our body will first use the stored energy from the liver and muscles for immediate energy, then when this is depleted, it will use the stored glucose in our fats cells through a process called gluconeogenesis. As we are physically active and require energy, our body uses our stored fat. If we eat more food than we require based on our physical activity and metabolism, we will store this excess as fat cells.

Our body is a delicate balance but extremely efficient in using the food we provide it. It was designed to need vitamins, minerals, phytonutrients and fibre that Mother Nature provides, and our cells are reliant on these nutrients for optimal health. Our brain, immune system, reproductive system, skeletal structure, lymphatic system, nervous system, respiratory system, cardiovascular system; in fact, our whole body cannot function without them.

Calories

A calorie is basically the amount of energy released when we digest and absorb a food or drink. We all understand that we burn calories while exercising, but we also use calories for breathing, digestion, movement, to keep our brain and organs functioning optimally, growing, healing, and to keep warm. This constant use of calories is called our metabolism.

We do not actually need that many calories to maintain our body's needs. Most adults only need between 1,500 and 2,000 calories, where children are growing and their caloric needs change as they age.

Approximate calories are:

2-3-year-old	1,000
4–8-year-old girl	1,200
4–8-year-old boy	1,400
9–13-year-old girl	1,600
9–13-year-old boy	1,800
14–18-year-old girl	1,800
14–18-year-old boy	2,200

The problem is that children are being exposed to foods that are very high in calories and a greater amount of it. For example, the calories in an apple are approximately fifty-six while the calories of two chocolate chip cookies are two hundred and fifty-six. There are around five hundred and seventy calories in two slices of pizza while only two hundred and seventy-one calories in a cup of vegetable stir-fry. A constant diet of highly caloric food will cause weight gain and health issues in children.

But weight gain isn't the only issue which must be addressed; what happens when we eat highly processed high sugar content food instead of the nutrient rich food that our body require? Highly processed high sugar foods will cause a spike in insulin and is usually followed by a crash of energy that has the person reaching for more sugar foods to give them the next energy boost. Constantly high insulin levels can create insulin resistance, which is where the cells become resistant to the insulin and the pancreas creates more insulin to try and get the glucose into the cells. If the pancreas wears out and can no longer produce enough insulin, the child is now diabetic and requires insulin injections.

These processed foods also contain high amounts of sodium, artificial flavouring, colouring, and saturated fats. Researchers are just discovering some of the damage that these foods are doing to our body, including non-alcoholic fatty liver disease, heart disease, cancer, and kidney disease. Try to limit these foods as much as you can and focus on providing natural whole foods in the home.

As parents, we are responsible for the health of our children, and ensuring that they eat a varied diet of natural healthy food is the best way we can ensure optimal health, growth, and wellbeing. Vary the types of fruits, berries, vegetables, nuts, and seeds, to ensure that your child is consuming all the minerals, vitamins, phytonutrients, and fiber they require. Reduce animal source protein to a reasonable amount (which will also save you money) and supplement this with other sources of protein. Ensure they drink enough water to stay hydrated.

Many kids are fussy eaters and according to the Pennsylvania State University 93% of kids do not eat enough vegetables and 60% don't eat enough fruit. As you now know, plant foods are essential to a healthy body. Sometimes, as parents, we need to be creative in ensuring our children eat the foods they need.

When my daughter was around four years old, she went through a phase where she would only eat pasta, so I added lightly steamed vegetables to every pasta dish she ate. Broccoli, cauliflower, peas, peppers, beans, and carrots – I snuck vegetables into everything. Then she watched *The Land Before Time* (a children's dinosaur movie) and pretended she was a dinosaur, so I snuck in leafy greens (we called them leaves) and broccoli (trees) because that is what dinosaurs ate. Hey, as a parent, you have to work with what you have.

Sometimes changing the way a food is cooked (baked, steamed, broiled, or raw) can help overcome objections, and I recommend you try different types of vegetables, add them to every dish you serve and don't give up if they refuse it the first time.

Older kids are a bit trickier, but I found that green smoothies, wraps loaded with leafy greens and vegetables as well as serving three different vegetables with dinner seemed to do the trick. They are probably going to eat processed foods outside of the home but if you can provide them the healthiest options for at-home meals, it will provide them with a foundation of health.

Recipe: Crunchy Snack

Roasted chickpeas are a great source of protein and fibre, and it gives a satisfying crunch like a potato chip. They are easy to make, and you have the option to pick your favourite seasonings.

Ingredients

1 can chickpeas (garbanzo beans)
2 tsp extra virgin olive oil
Dash salt
1 tsp garlic powder
¼ cup diced green onions.
(Option: use 1 tsp onion salt in place of salt and green onions)

Preheat oven to 375 degrees. Drain and rinse the chickpeas and layer in a baking sheet. Pat them dry with paper towel (the drier the better).

Bake 30-35 minutes shaking every ten minutes to prevent sticking. They should be golden brown and crunchy. Watch carefully so they don't burn.

In medium bowl, combine the salt, garlic powder and green onions.

Remove chickpeas from oven and immediately toss with olive oil then in seasonings. Cool before serving.

Tip:

If you have leftovers, store in an airtight container and roast again for ten minutes to re-crisp.

Chapter Fourteen: Portion Sizes

"Go vegetable heavy. Reverse the psychology of your plate by making meat the side dish and vegetables the main course."

-Bobby Flay

14

I would love to tell you exactly how many portions you should be feeding your child, but the number of portions are dependent on the age of the child, their size, activity, and growing periods. For this reason, I have recommended number of portions, but you will need to adjust based on your child's needs. I recommend you provide smaller portions and then extra helpings if they are still hungry. It takes time for our brain to signal our body that we have had enough food, and eating slower with smaller portions is the best way to know if we are full without overeating.

You may notice that the suggested number of portions in this book do not match with the Food Pyramid or My Plate from Canada that you may be familiar with. While I think the governments are making progress, I have a problem with the current recommended number of servings because their program is still heavily influenced by big business and not by the best nutritional health. Let me explain a bit more.

If you want to keep a cow or goat lean, farmers let it graze on grass, leaves and other vegetable sources of food. But, if the farmer wants to fatten up the animal for slaughter, the animal is fed high amounts of grains. The recommended food pyramid/plate is, in my opinion, too high in grains. This can cause weight gain; and since most people use bread as their grain option (which has low quality fats, processed sugar and wheat) rather than natural grains, it has an even worse effect.

While they have added milk alternatives, and other sources of non-animal protein, there is still a push for a higher amount of animal protein than is necessary for optimal health. Multiple scientific studies, including the famous China Project, as well as real-life examples during World War Two when meat was not available, have all shown that eating less meat and eating more natural vegetables, fruits and berries can improve the overall health of the public.

The China Project (sometimes called the China Study) was completed in the early 1980's by Cornell University, Oxford University and the Chinese Academy of Preventive Medicine. Sixty-five counties in rural China were selected for the study of diet, disease and lifestyle characteristics for a total of 6500 participants. In 1989, twenty new counties in mainland China and Taiwan were added to bring the total to 10'200 participants. The results of this massive study clearly demonstrated that people who ate a mainly plant based diet had few or no chronic diseases, while those who ate high amounts of animal meat had the most chronic disease, including cancer, heart disease and diabetes.

During World War II, the Germans confiscated all of the livestock from the Norwegian countries they occupied in order to feed their own troops. This forced vegetarianism of the local population caused deaths from strokes and heart attacks to be drastically reduced and when animal protein was reintroduced at the end of the war, the rates of heart disease rose dramatically to pre-war levels.

I am not telling you to become a vegetarian, but I am saying that promoting high levels of animal protein in our food pyramid is not in our best health interest. Promoting plant-based protein sources should be a higher priority if the overall health of the population is the main objective.

I know that dairy farmers, cattle farmers and grain farmers have all influenced the decision of governments in their dietary recommendations to the public, and I understand why, but my recommendations to you have been adjusted for optimal health. Unlike these business-oriented groups and government agencies, my first priority is to provide you with the best health solutions.

When introducing a new food to a toddler, sometimes they are fussy and do not want to eat a particular food but may accept it at a later time, so don't give up too easily as it takes multiple exposures to a specific food before a child accepts it. There will be days where they love a particular food and want it with every meal and then a week later (usually after you have stocked up on it) they decide they no longer like it.

Young children also have more taste buds than adults, so a food may seem too bitter, salty, or spicy for them even if it tastes fine for us, so keep food a bit blander. Serve fresh vegetables, berries, whole grains, lean protein, and fruit and try not to serve food that is high in added sugars, preservatives, or food additives. Limit deep-fried foods and processed snack foods, so they eat more natural foods. I know this sounds like a lot of work to you because you are a busy parent, but this will create a healthy eating pattern for your child all their life.

There is a theory that children who are exposed to processed sugar foods (such as cookies, ice cream etc.) at a young age have a change in the development of their taste buds and brain receptors. These changes encourage them to crave more sweet foods. You may have heard the term 'having a sweet tooth,' for when a person craves sugar sweetened foods. Young children are more affected by processed sugar due to their size and metabolism and these foods should be avoided as much as possible. Please note that I am talking about processed sugar, not the natural sugar of whole fruit or berries.

The first solid food is not eaten before six months of age when the digestive tract immunological systems have developed to reduce the possibility of allergy or other reactions to food. First foods should be natural, simple, without sugar, pureed and easy to digest. Pureed cooked fruit such as apples, pears, plums, or cooked and pureed vegetables (yams and squash work well) and cooked cereal grains. These foods, along with mother's milk or formula, provide the nutrition needed. Once the teeth start to appear at around eight months, you can add in cooked potatoes, broccoli, meat, and eggs. Be aware some children have egg allergies, so watch them carefully whenever you are introducing a new food.

Parents often overestimate the amount of food needed, so keep meals simple and serve smaller portions more frequently throughout the day. Toddlers are exceptionally good at knowing when they have had enough to eat, and you should never shove food in their mouth to force them to eat more. They will give you cues such as turning their head away, gagging, crying, spitting out the food, or trying to leave the table. My granddaughter says, "All done" and tries to hand me the plate. Sometimes I am fast enough to catch it, but sometimes I am not quick enough, and the food ends up on the floor. Children know when they have had enough food and are not afraid to tell you.

Never force a child to finish what is on their plate; as adults, we often give too much and worry they are not eating enough. Aim to give one tablespoon of food per year of age for each meal. For example, a three-year-old would receive three tablespoons of food for the meal. If they want more, they will let you know. Serve healthy snacks in between mealtimes rather than having the child eat only three meals a day. Most young children are grazers by nature, and although we may worry they are not eating enough, they will consume enough food throughout the day.

Toddlers should not have more than ½ a cup of fruit juice a day and I recommend watering it down so there is less sweetness to it. Juice should never be left in a bottle in the crib or out for them to sip on over a longer period as this will promote tooth decay. If you choose to give them juice, serve it at the table and remove it when they are done. After twelve months of age, encourage your little ones to drink water in between meals and snacks to create healthy habits for life.

For children ages four to five, aim to provide three servings of vegetables, two servings of fruit or berries, one servings of processed grains, one serving of unprocessed grains, two servings of milk or alternatives and two servings of meat or alternatives throughout the day. This food should be served as three meals and three snacks (please note that some children do not require an evening snack). You may offer ¼ cup of nuts and seeds (not peanuts due to allergies and mold), but only if there is no risk of choking. Also be sure to always watch for allergies. For example, you could choose to serve

- Breakfast: oatmeal with side of blueberries, water
- Snack: sliced apple with walnuts

- Lunch: ½ chicken sandwich with glass of milk
- Snack: carrot sticks and dip, water
- Dinner: mashed potatoes, steamed broccoli and meatloaf, water
- Snack: glass of milk

Ages six to eight will have three servings of vegetables, one serving of leafy greens, two servings of fruit or berries, one serving of processed grains, one serving of unprocessed grains, two servings of milk or alternatives, two servings of protein, and one serving of nuts and seeds. For example, you could serve:

- Breakfast: Plain Cheerios with blueberries
- Morning Snack: Apple with almonds
- Lunch: Turkey sandwich with carrot sticks
- Afternoon Snack: Cucumbers and bell peppers
- Dinner: Fish, steamed broccoli, brown rice, beets, glass of milk.

From ages nine to eleven, increase vegetables to four servings, one serving leafy greens, two servings of fruit or berries, two servings of processed grains, one serving unprocessed grains, two servings of milk or alternatives, one to two servings of protein, and one serving of nuts and seeds.

To translate these portions into real food, you could serve a nine-year-old:

- Breakfast: Oatmeal with berries, glass of milk

- Lunch: Whole-wheat wrap with chicken and one cup of sliced peppers, onions, lettuce.
- Snack: Baby carrots and orange
- Dinner: Pork chop, brown rice, broccoli, cauliflower, peas, glass of milk.

While physical growth slows a bit from four to twelve years of age, the mental growth is relatively rapid. This is a perfect time to instill healthy eating habits by encouraging the consumption of quality whole natural foods. Kids at this age look to you as an example, so eating healthy foods together as a family will go a long way to creating a great foundation.

Start teaching them how to shop for food, how to prepare food and help them to learn about the various food options. They can begin to help prepare their school lunches and after school snacks. Encourage them to try new fruits and vegetables and help them pick out new food at the grocery store for the family to try.

After the age of twelve, your child will have their own food preferences and the number of portions will vary depending on their gender, height, body size, activity level, and whether they are in a growth period. Aim to provide two to three servings of fruit or berries, four servings of vegetables, two leafy greens, two servings of processed grains, two servings of unprocessed grains, one serving of nuts and seeds, two servings of protein, and two servings of milk or alternatives. Teenagers also need a lot of water! For example, you could serve:

- Breakfast: Oatmeal with berries
- Lunch: Chicken sandwich with lettuce, apple, raw carrots and snap peas, glass of milk or alternative.

- Snack: Banana, mixed nuts, raw vegetables with dip
- Dinner: Meatloaf, peas, cauliflower and side salad with glass of milk or alternative.

Avoid serving any sugary drinks, flavored milk, energy drinks, sports drinks, and soda. An active teenager in a growth period can eat an enormous amount of food, so having apples, bananas and oranges for snacks and a big salad at dinner is a great way to help satisfy their seemingly never-ending hunger and still provide nutrition.

Kids love snacks, whether mid-day or after school or during a movie or before bed. When changing the type of snacks for your family, the trick is to offer a variety of healthy snacks that do not make anyone feel deprived. If you ban a particular food, then chances are they will crave it, hide it, or binge eat when they are allowed the food. If your child loves a particular snack food which is less than healthy, purchase it less often (such as during the once-a-month free day) and in smaller portion sizes. All things in moderation.

Healthy snack options include:

- Fresh fruit.
- Berries.
- Nuts.
- Seeds.
- Air popped popcorn with unsalted butter.
- Plain full fat yogurt (add the berries for a bit of sweetness if you desire).
- Celery with nut butters.

- Plain oatmeal with added cinnamon and diced apples.
- Veggie pita pocket.
- Homemade fruit or berry smoothies.
- Hard-boiled eggs.
- Homemade baked sweet potato fries.
- Carrot sticks and hummus.
- Bell peppers and guacamole.
- Unsweetened applesauce pouches.

Offer a snack midmorning and afternoon for toddlers and children, and in the afternoon for pre-teens and teenagers. Kids can come home ravenous and the first thing they do is open the fridge door and yell 'what's there to eat?' and they will reach for the first thing to fill an empty stomach. Be prepared with healthy food on hand.

Keep fruit on the table or counter for easy access. Put berries, cut melons, vegetables, and healthy dips at eye level in the fridge so they are more likely to reach for those. In my house, I found that if I cut up a melon and put it in a bowl in the fridge, it would be eaten, but if I left it whole, then no one would touch it. If you do have cookies, crackers, chips, or similar foods in the house, tuck them away in a cupboard so they are not as obvious. Have a jug of cold unsweetened tea or milk for them to drink rather than soda or fruit juice (because there is little fiber in fruit juice, and it is extremely high in sugar).

Continuous snacking can interfere with food consumption during a meal. So, it is important to keep snacking to specific times of the day in order to avoid this. Some kids (especially young ones) seem to snack or graze all day long. For young children up to the age of twelve, offer breakfast, a mid-morning snack, two to three hours after breakfast, lunch then another snack, three hours after lunch, then dinner. You can offer a bedtime snack if they are really hungry, but otherwise avoid feeding them right before bed since it can interfere with digestion and sleep habits. Older children do not need the midmorning snack but may still require a snack after school.

Kids should eat at the table whether it is a meal or snacks (which also keeps the mess to a minimum in the rest of the house), as this teaches them to eat their food without distractions. Let them focus on the taste, smell, and appearance of the food and avoid overeating or mindless eating. When we eat while watching television, reading or doing other activities, we are not aware of how much we are eating, eat much larger amounts, and is the main cause of binge eating. Turn off the television, phones, computers and other distractions and let them focus on creating healthy eating habits.

Water should be served at snack time instead of juice, soda, or energy drinks, as kids are busy and can become dehydrated easily. Thirst can be confused for hunger, so drinking water can help them avoid empty caloric snacks. Water is essential for life and kids should get in the habit of drinking water instead of sugary drinks.

A Harvard University study found that fifty percent of children were chronically dehydrated due to inadequate water intake, as well as insufficient fresh fruits and vegetables. Water satiates the body, is essential to life and free from the tap, which helps you save money on your food budget.

Toddlers and small children have a higher body water percentage, metabolic rates and turnover of fluids in their body. This means that they have an increased risk of dehydration and drinking water with meals and snacks should be encouraged.

Teenage years can be a period of nutritional risk because parents have less control over their eating habits. Peer pressure is huge and so is the impact of the media. They may tend to eat a lot of refined foods, sweets, soda, fast food, and processed foods when they are away from home. The best you can do is to encourage them to eat healthy and provide healthy food and snacks at home for their dinner and breakfast meals.

Caloric needs are higher during this time, as they are growing physically and mentally and may be busy with sports or other activities. You may also wish to speak with their doctor about adding in a vitamin and mineral supplement (especially for girls who begin menstruation) to their daily regime. Our food is becoming less nutritious due to depleted soil; hence, a multivitamin can help supplement this.

Serving Size Summary

Fruits, berries, melons, and vegetables

Fresh, frozen, or canned vegetables
125 mL (½ cup)
Leafy vegetables
250 mL (1 cup)
Fresh, frozen, or canned fruits, berries, melons
1 fruit or 125 mL (½ cup)
100% Juice
125 mL (½ cup)

Processed carbohydrates/grains

Bread
1 slice (35 g)
Bagel (small size. Note Tim Horton's bagels are large).
½ bagel (45 g)
Flat breads
½ pita or ½ tortilla (35 g)
Cooked pasta or couscous 125 mL (½ cup)

Boxed Cereal
Cold: 30 g or ¼ cup

Unprocessed grains

Cooked rice, bulgur, or quinoa
125 mL (½ cup)
Cooked cereal: 175 mL (¾ cup)

Milk and alternatives

Cow milk, almond milk
250 mL (1 cup)
Canned milk (evaporated)
125 mL (½ cup)
Fortified soy beverage
250 mL (1 cup)
Yogurt
175 g (¾ cup)
Cheese
50 g (1/4 cup or 1 ½ oz.)

Meat and alternatives

Cooked fish, shellfish, poultry, lean meat
75 g (2 ½ oz.) or 125 mL (½ cup) or size of deck of cards
Cooked legumes
175 mL (3/4 cup)
Tofu
150 g or 175 mL (¾ cup)
Eggs
2 eggs
Peanut or nut butters
30 mL (2 Tbsp)
Shelled nuts and seeds
60 mL (¼ cup)

Oils and fats

Healthy oil (canola, olive, soybean)
30 to 45 mL or 2 to 3 tbsp

On the next page, you will find a Daily Recommended Intake (DRI) of nutrients for children from age 1-18. These numbers are for the total intake including food, and are an approximate because there are height, weight, activity level, muscularity and health differences that are unique to each child. You can use these as a general guide to determine if they are obtaining enough nutrients.

You will note that iron is different during menstruation. Iron supplements are best taken on a full stomach, or they can cause nausea. If you choose to take a liquid iron supplement, which is easier to absorb, be aware that it can cause staining of the teeth. Your child can drink it through a straw to try and avoid the front teeth. If they must take the liquid form, dilute it with water, and make sure to rinse the mouth immediately and brush teeth after fifteen minutes.

Tracking a child's daily intake of nutrients can be very difficult. There are several online free food trackers (MyPlate, MyFitnessPal, Cronometer) that can track calories, protein, carbohydrates, fats, vitamins and minerals. However, what you give them may not actually be what they eat. For instance, you can give your child one medium apple, but they may avoid the brown spot, won't eat near the core and end up giving half to the dog. Unless you are spoon-feeding them, all you will get are estimates but that is okay. Just do the best you can. I created *My Health Tracker for Kids* (available on Amazon) which is a portion styled health tracker, that can help you to ensure they are receiving enough variety and the correct number of portions but will not track the individual vitamins or minerals.

Daily Recommended Intake

Nutrient	Age 1-3 Yrs	Age 4-8	Age 9-13	Age 14-18
Calories	1000-1400	1600-2000	2000-2400	3150/girls2000-2400
Protein	1.2/kg	30-35 g	35-45 g	boys 56g/girls46 g
Vitamin A	2000 IU	3000 IU	4000 IU	5400 IU
Vitamin D	400 IU	400 IU	400 IU	300 IU
Vitamin E	8 IU	20 IU	25 IU	30 IU
Vitamin K	30 mcg	55 mcg	60 mcg	150 mcg
Thiamin (B1)	0.8 mg	1.0 mg	1.5 mg	1.5 mg
Riboflavin (B2)	0.9 mg	1.2 mg	1.6 mg	2 mg
Niacin (B3)	10 mg	12 mg	17 mg	18 mg
Pantothenic acid (B5)	4 mg	4 mg	5 mg	10 mg
Pyridoxine (B6)	1.0 mg	1.5 mg	2.0 mg	2.5 mg
Cobalamin (B12)	2.5 mcg	3 mcg	4 mcg	5 mcg
Folic acid	150 mcg	250 mcg	350 mcg	400 mcg
Biotin	16 mcg	25 mcg	50 mcg	200 mcg
Vitamin C	100mg	75 mg	135 mg	300 mg
Calcium	800 mg	800 mg	1300 mg	1200 mg
Chloride	1.2 g	1.5 g	2.0 g	3.0 g
Chromium	80 mcg	45 mcg	75 mcg	200 mcg
Copper	0.6 mg	0.8 mg	1.4 mg	2-3 mg
Fluoride	1.0 mg	2.0 mg	2.5 mg	2.5 mg
Iodine	190 mcg	120 mcg	120 mcg	150 mcg
Iron	10 mg girl	10 mg girl	8 mg girl	menstruating/11mg not menstruating
	10 mg boy	10 mg boy	8 mg boy	11 mg boy
Magnesium	150 mg	250 mg	300 mg	400 mg
Manganese	1.5 mg	2.5 mg	3.0 mg	5 mg
Molybdenum	40 mcg	50 mcg	75 mcg	100 mcg
Phosphorus	800 mg	800 mg	1250 mg	1200 mg
Potassium	1.5 mg	2.0 g	2.5 g	4 g
Selenium	80 mcg	90 mcg	120 mcg	200 mcg
Sodium	0.9 g	1.3 g	1.8 g	3 g
Zinc	10 mg	10 mg	16 mg	15 mg

Common Sources of Nutrients

(Please note that this list is not exhaustive or in order of percentage of the nutrient. This list offers a general knowledge).

Nutrient	Common Sources
Protein	Animal, Fish, Poultry, Plant sources, dairy
Vitamin A	Leafy green vegetables, orange vegetables, fish oils
Vitamin D	Eggs, oily fish, oysters, liver, milk, almond milk, tofu
Vitamin E	Sunflower seeds, pumpkin, red bell pepper, spinach, avocado, wheat germ oil, almonds
Vitamin K	Cabbage, Brussel sprouts, Broccoli, Kiwi, Asparagus, Leafy greens, blueberries, egg, carrots
Thiamin (B1)	Egg, fish, lentils, brown rice, sunflower seed, legume, orange, green peas, chicken, mussels
Riboflavin (B2)	Egg, beef, sweet potatoes, almonds, dairy products, leafy vegetables, chicken, lentils, pork
Niacin (B3)	Egg, fish, chicken, turkey, brown rice, sunflower seed, spinach, avocado, potatoes, milk
Pantothenic acid (B5)	Organ meats, chicken, beef, mushrooms, avocado, nuts, seeds, dairy, eggs, brown rice
Pyridoxine (B6)	Eggs, banana, spinach, chickpea, fish, chicken, pork, lentils, beans, carrots, sunflower seed

Cobalamin (B12)	Beef liver, tuna, salmon, eggs, turkey, tempeh, banana, strawberries, whole wheat bread
Folic acid	Dark green leafy vegetables, broccoli, beans, whole grains, sunflower seeds, eggs, fresh fruit
Biotin	Eggs, organ meats, legumes, mushrooms, sweet potato, avocado, spinach, cauliflower, oats
Vitamin C	Citrus fruits, red and green peppers, broccoli, strawberries, Brussel sprouts, cantaloupe
Calcium	Dairy, edamame, tofu, winter squash, almonds, dark green leafy vegetables, figs, canned salmon
Chloride	Seaweed, rye, tomatoes, lettuce, celery, olives, table salt, barley, potatoes
Chromium	Eggs, green beans, broccoli, whole grains, banana, fish, barley, turkey, Brazil nuts, apple, tomato
Copper	Cashews, leafy greens, oysters, dark chocolate, chickpeas, quinoa, spirulina, sunflower seeds
Fluoride	Canned shellfish, oatmeal, raisins, potatoes,
Iodine	Prunes, fish, dairy, navy beans, oysters, banana, iodized salt, cheese, nori
Iron	Red meat, lentils, spinach, chickpea, oysters, cashews, quinoa, beans, eggs, leafy vegetables, turkey
Magnesium	Pumpkin seeds, leafy vegetables, almonds, bananas, avocado, fish, whole grains, chia seeds

Manganese	Clams, oysters, mussels, leafy greens, brown rice, oatmeal, legumes
Molybdenum	Legumes, whole grains, nuts, eggs, beef, chicken, rice, potatoes, nuts
Phosphorus	Dairy products, fish, meat, poultry, eggs, legumes, nuts, oatmeal, bran, beans, lentils
Potassium	Bananas, beet greens, avocado, winter squash, potatoes, beans, lentils, sweet potatoes
Selenium	Brazil nuts, organ meats, seafood, banana, dairy, white button or shiitake mushrooms,
Sodium	Canned vegetables, olives, pickles, apples, avocados, banana, pears, celery, spinach, carrots
Zinc	Meat, fish, seafood, pomegranate, raspberries, guava, mushrooms, spinach, kale, garlic, broccoli

Chapter Fifteen: Easy Swaps for Better Health

"Healthy eating isn't about counting fat grams, dieting, cleanses, and antioxidants; it's about eating food untouched from the way we find it in nature in a balanced way."
-Pooja Mottl

15

You may have the best of intentions to eat healthy natural food prepared by you at every meal, but let's be honest, you are busy and there will be times when you are going to buy a pre-made, not so healthy food, especially if it is a family favourite. Pre-made healthy foods can be pricey, and the average family is on a limited food budget, but there are ways to make each meal a bit healthier for the whole family.

Add vegetables to everything. Seriously! This is the easiest and quickest way to better health. If you bought a frozen pepperoni pizza for dinner, then add tiny pieces of peppers and mushrooms and serve it with a side salad. If you are having instant soup, add fresh or frozen vegetables to improve the meal. Add lettuce, tomato, onion and avocado to a burger and tiny pieces of carrot, celery, onion and spinach to meatloaf. Think of ways that you can add more vegetables to the meals you are currently preparing.

Change the side dishes at your favourite restaurant to a side salad, raw or steamed vegetables, or coleslaw and avoid the highly caloric breadbasket, French fries or tortilla chips. The average side of French fries in a restaurant contains five hundred calories plus if you add ketchup, it can be over six hundred. Also, be aware that many store-bought salad dressings contain an extremely high amount of salt, saturated fat and sugar. So, limit the amount of dressing or make your own healthier version if you are eating at home. For some great online recipes, look at diabetic websites, as they usually have the healthier and tastier options.

The way we prepare food can also make a big difference in the quality of the meal. For example, instead of deep-frying in oil, bake chicken in an air fryer or convection oven to reduce the oil used in preparation. Avoid using breading or batter on foods and use herbs and spices instead. Changing the way we cook foods can save hundreds of calories and reduce the amount of saturated fats we consume, which contribute to high blood pressure and heart disease.

Serve pasta as a side dish instead of the main entrée or substitute the white pasta for baked spaghetti squash or zucchini. White pasta is a highly refined carbohydrate that can increase our sugar levels very quickly. By serving a smaller portion or swapping it out for a vegetable, we will reduce our glucose and insulin levels. Also, add loads of vegetables such as peppers, onions, garlic, and celery to your sauce to increase your vegetables and reduce the glycemic load of the meal.

Have clear broth soups instead of cream-based soups. Many soups are made with heavy cream, which is much higher in saturated fat and sodium than a clear-based soup. You can make a large batch of vegetable-based soup and freeze extra portions for a quick nutritious meal later on.

Pre-make green smoothies with their favourite fruits (you don't taste the greens because of the fruit) and add chia or ground flaxseed for healthy fats. These smoothies can be kept in the fridge for several days or frozen, and are a great after school snack, or an on the run breakfast. I should warn you; if you make a smoothie with strawberries and leafy greens, or blueberries and leafy greens it will go a sort of brown colour. It tastes great, but the colour may be off putting to some people. I included the recipe in the book for your convenience.

Change to a healthier breakfast cereal. Many breakfast cereals have more sugar per serving than a candy bar and no one eats the recommended serving size. By switching to a lower sugar content cereal, you can reduce the amount of sugar your kids are eating. Read the labels on the side of the box and look for at least three grams of fiber and less than six grams of sugar per serving. One trick I used to do when my daughter was young was to mix plain Cheerios with the Honey Nut Cheerios in order to reduce the amount of sugar she was consuming. She got her favourite cereal, and I knew she was eating less sugar. A win for both of us!

Switch from white rice to brown or wild rice. White rice has a higher glycemic index, meaning it converts into glucose much faster and creates a spike in insulin. Now, not everyone likes the taste or texture of brown rice, but it is much healthier as it still contains the bran and germ of the grain, and digests slower which keeps insulin levels lower. When I was changing from white to brown rice, I would mix the two types of rice when I prepared it, and gradually reduced the percentage of white rice until they were eating only brown rice.

Limit sugary drinks and encourage children to drink more water. Children should not be drinking soda on a regular basis as it increases the risk of obesity, dental cavities, fatty liver disease, and kidney disease. A child size Coca-Cola from McDonalds has one-hundred calories and twenty-six grams of sugar. We don't realize how those sports drinks, energy drinks and fancy drinks from Starbucks, Tim Hortons and McDonald's add up our total caloric intake. I realize these drinks are very popular with teenagers, but if your body needs only fifteen hundred calories a day and your Mocha Frappuccino has five hundred calories (caloric number provided by Starbucks), then it leaves you with only one thousand calories for food. These drinks provide no nutrition, fiber or help to the body, but they do provide a high amount of sugar, artificial colouring, and flavouring which have a greater effect on children.

Switch them to drinking whole milk (depending on the age of the child), or water. They may complain about not having their favourite soda or fruit juice in the house, but they will adapt. When they are young, most children are able to drink milk as they have a greater number of lactase enzymes, which allow them to digest milk more easily. They should drink whole milk and not a lower fat such as two percent because they need the fat for growth. As they get older (usually in the teens), levels of lactase start to drop, and some children may start having issues with milk and milk products and can switch to milk alternatives or water.

Some other easy swaps for better health are:

• Encourage them to eat fresh whole fruits such as apples, bananas, or oranges (buy fruits in season to lower the cost) instead of cookies, crackers, or pretzels. Whole fruit contains natural fibre, which slows the absorption of the fructose and provides vitamins and minerals.
• Switch from white bread to whole grain. White bread is made from highly processed flour, with the germ and bran removed from the grain leaving it with no

fibre, and a high glycemic index that raises insulin levels.

- For lunch, have vegetable soup or a wrap made with vegetables, leafy greens, and sprouts instead of a sandwich. Adding more vegetables provide greater nutrients and fibre in the meal.

- Have them eat eggs or oatmeal for breakfast instead of boxed cereal. Eggs with vegetables such as peppers, mushrooms, onions, and spinach provide an excellent source of lean protein, vitamins and minerals that are low glycemic and provides long lasting energy. Oatmeal with berries provides a great source of slow digesting fibre, antioxidants, phytonutrients, vitamins, and minerals that will keep your child feeling full much longer than boxed cereals.

- Serve fresh cut vegetables and dip instead of potato chips or pretzels.

- If you are serving potato chips, provide a smaller portion - not individual bags.

- Purchase salt free products such as tomato sauce, soups, or canned vegetables.

- Most condiments contain high amounts of sugar, salt, and saturated fats. Use mustard instead of mayonnaise, and skip the barbeque sauce, ketchup, and other high sugar content sauces. Try using herbs and spices instead of added sauces or dips.

- Eat leaner cuts of meat and fish and avoid processed meats (such as bologna, salami, bacon, pepperoni, and chicken nuggets), which are high in saturated fats, salt, nitrates, additives, and preservatives.

Children can be suspicious of new foods and will often say they don't like it, even when they have never tried it. When introducing new healthy foods, try mixing them with the foods they eat and enjoy currently. For example, add lightly steamed broccoli to macaroni and cheese, add extra vegetables to a soup or stew, add carrots to meat loaf, or raw vegetables with a homemade dipping sauce.

Encourage children to try new types of fruits and vegetables by allowing them to select a new food from the grocery store or helping you prepare the food. Children will be more enthusiastic for something that they choose over something that is seemingly forced upon them. My granddaughter would not eat tomatoes until she helped me to grow cherry tomatoes in the garden and now she eats them all the time.

Making these changes all at once can be overwhelming, so start with two or three healthy swaps at a time. For example, stop buying fruit juice or soda and buy whole fruit instead. Make them oatmeal with berries or scrambled eggs with vegetables instead of giving them a sugary-boxed cereal. Serve raw vegetables and dip on movie nights instead of chips. Stop buying pop tarts and cookies and put a fruit bowl on the table.

Depending on the age of the child, you can create a healthier lifestyle plan together. Make sure you listen to their ideas and incorporate some of them into your plan. This will create 'buy in' and will make your child want to participate more. Let them choose a new fruit or vegetable from the grocery store. Look up healthy recipes together and teach them how to cook. If you don't know how to cook, why not take a cooking class together? Incorporate foods that they enjoy in your menu planning and talk to them about fun activities they want to include in your new lifestyle.

Please be aware that your child may have anxiety or fears about changing to a healthier lifestyle, such as having to give up their favourite foods or that they will never be able to have a birthday party with their friends again. Talk to them about having a healthy balance in life and what they will look like in your home. No one knows your child like you do and you know the best way to make changes in your home without causing unnecessary stress and anxiety.

Recipe: Avocado Toast

Ingredients:

2 slices whole grain or rye toast
2 eggs poached or sunny side up
¼ avocado mashed
Salt & pepper to taste
Sprinkle of chilli powder or cayenne pepper if you prefer.

Toast bread and prepare eggs to your liking.

Spread mashed avocado on toast. Add sprinkle of chilli powder.

Add eggs. Salt & pepper to taste.

Tip:

Do not use frozen avocado, fresh only.

Chapter Sixteen: Saving Time and Money

"Cutting food waste is a delicious way of saving money, helping to feed the world and protect the planet."

-Tristram Stuart

16

Did you know that families that use menu planning are more likely to stick to their new healthy lifestyle, eat nutritious food, eat vegetables, salads and fruits, eat a more varied diet, spend less money on their food budget, and experience greater weight loss and improved health. Sounds great, doesn't it?

I'm not going to lie to you, in the beginning, it takes thought and effort to plan out meals and do bulk cooking, but easier to slip back into old habits. This is why menu planning can be very helpful, as it helps to keep us on track because when we know what the plan is, we don't reach for those last-minute 'quick, I need to get supper on the table' foods that got us into trouble in the first place.

When I am working with clients, we create a menu that includes breakfast, lunch, supper and one snack. If they have toddlers or grade school children, we may include two snacks. My clients choose foods they can either make in bulk or have time to cook during the week, foods they like and can afford. We work on a menu that has planned leftovers for either lunch or dinner the next day. If they have older children, they should allow them to contribute ideas to the menu, so they feel a part of the solution and are more encouraged to stick to the plan.

Once the menu is created, it is posted on the fridge for everyone to see. This also allows all the adults and older children to be able to help to prep and cook meals, instead of dumping everything on the parent. No more excuses of 'but I didn't know what you want to make for dinner, so I didn't start anything.' Younger children can help to set the table and put out water glasses.

People tend to associate meal planning with a rigid structure that they must adhere to, but it doesn't have to be like that. You can create a menu for a week that has flexibility built into it for last minute events, or work schedules. I also like to plan a 'free' day once a month that allows family members to eat their 'less than healthy foods.' This helps to avoid intense cravings that may cause them to stop following a healthy dietary plan. When we have a built-in free day, we don't feel deprived because we know we are going to have that old favourite food once a month.

To start your menu planning, I recommend that you scan the grocery store flyers, create your plan based on what is in season and on sale at the time, then write out your grocery list and attach any coupons to it. Have something to eat (because you never want to go to the grocery store hungry), then do your shopping. Stick to your list! Unless you have forgotten something major, like toilet paper, if it isn't on your list, then don't buy it and don't fall for the 'but it is on sale' trap that makes us buy extra food.

When you return home, wash and prep your fruits and vegetables right away, so they don't turn into those mushy science experiments in the bottom drawer of the fridge. You may decide to cook some of your meals for the week on this day as well so you can save time later on. Older kids can help with these tasks to teach them healthy lifestyle skills and to reduce the amount of work for you.

Once healthy eating becomes a habit, you won't have to create menus or work as hard at this. But I'm not going to lie to you, in the beginning, it takes work, and you will slip up from time to time. Keep going! I have faith that you will adapt to your healthy lifestyle very quickly. Once you start, you may even find that menu planning saves you so much time and money that you continue doing it.

I often hear that natural whole food is more expensive than convenient processed foods and I agree, but there are ways to stick to your budget and eat healthy. Avoiding food waste is easier when you plan out your meals. The average American family throws out $1600 per year in produce and, overall, Americans waste $218 billion on food (Food Waste in America 2023). According to Statistics Canada, Canadians waste 50 million tonnes of food each year.

We have all bought food with the best intention of eating it only to forget it in the fridge. Or we make a meal and think we will eat the leftovers the next day but end up going out for our meal and the leftovers are thrown away, wasting food and money. In addition, take-out food is not re-utilized the way other foods are. For example, if you have French fries and couldn't eat them all, you probably won't be able to reuse them the next day, while if you cooked potatoes, you could reuse them in soups, stews, fried potatoes etc.

Some grocery stores are more expensive than others, so consider shopping at a different store to get a better deal. Use store brands or generic as they are often cheaper but made in the same factory as the more expensive brands.

Use coupons and store points to save money on future purchases but remember never to use a coupon for something you won't actually eat within the next week. If you can't resist buying a specific unhealthy food, don't go down that aisle in the grocery store. For me, the smell of the fresh baked bread makes me crave pie, cake and cookies. I intentionally avoid that section of the store to avoid temptation.

To avoid throwing away food, create intentional leftovers (for lunch or dinner the next day), or if you aren't a fan of leftovers, pick meals that can be repurposed, such as chicken that can be used in a tortilla or on a salad the next day. Leftover vegetables from dinner can easily be added to soups or pasta for a healthier more filling meal. Even instant dried soups, such as Mr. Noodle, can be healthier by adding vegetables.

Bulk cooking is your friend: If you are going to go to the trouble to bake a chicken breast, cook six, then freeze the extra and use them for stir-fry, sandwiches or on top of salad later on. You can even take the frozen meat in your lunch, and by mealtime, it will be defrosted, and you are able to add it to your salad. The same concept is true with soups, stews, and casseroles. Hard boil a dozen eggs and use them throughout the week. You can also make a large pot of oatmeal and then put it in individual containers that can be reheated later (I like adding frozen berries to mine, then heating it up for a healthy fruit cobbler).

Use a slow cooker to create meals by adding your choice of lean meat with vegetables to the pot in the morning and have it ready to eat when you get home.

Insta Pots are becoming very popular for cooking healthy foods faster.

If you don't have time to wash and cut up fresh vegetables, bagged and frozen are another great option. Bagged vegetables are a bit more expensive, but they can be helpful if time is your biggest concern. Flash frozen vegetables are minimally processed and are still a healthy option that can easily be added to canned soups, casseroles, stew or served as a side dish.

Make planned leftovers for lunch the next day by making a little extra for dinner, and then putting it in containers at the same time you are serving the meal. I found that this also helps to prevent eating too much or nibbling on the leftovers because there is none left to tempt me. Out of sight- out of mind. If your family enjoys second helpings, have a big salad and tell them they can eat more salad as the rest of the leftovers are for lunch tomorrow.

Make soups or stews that can be frozen and used later on. This is perfect for meals in a hurry. Bulk cooking saves time! If you are going to heat up the oven to cook four chicken drumsticks, why not cook a dozen and freeze the leftovers? If you are going to make a pot of soup, double the recipe and use the rest the next day or freeze it.

Remember, every meal or snack doesn't have to be fancy, and in fact, simple meals are easier and faster for most families. The internet has some great time saving ideas for healthy eating, so look online and decide what will work for your family. Choose something simple that your family will enjoy that is within your budget and time restraints.

The bulk food section can be a good option for dry goods such as rice, quinoa, oatmeal, nuts, seeds, legumes and spices, and are usually much cheaper than the individual containers. Swapping out white flour products for whole grain is an easy change at the same price.

Buy fresh local fruits and vegetables that are in season when you can. If you purchase grapes in winter, you can expect to pay a very high price, but apples or bananas may be a much cheaper option. Some vegetables, such as turnips, carrots, yams, cabbage and squash last much longer than others, so they don't go to waste in your fridge.

Add vegetarian options to your menu plan to lower the amount of animal products and fish, which are more expensive. Studies show that eating vegetarian is a very healthy option.

You may want to consider growing your own food in the backyard, community garden or even in a windowsill (if this is an option for you). In Canada, there are 6.2 million lawns, and converting just one quarter of each would produce over 14,000 hectares of gardens. In the United States, there are over forty million acres of lawn. Imagine how much food we could grow in this space. If you are going to do all the work and expense of watering, fertilizing, and mowing – why not grow something you can eat?

Some vegetables such as radish, lettuce, and spinach can grow in very small pots with limited light such as an apartment balcony. If you have a window with enough light, herbs are a great thing to grow to give your food more flavour and nutrition.

If you don't have the time or space for a garden, perhaps you know someone who does and is willing to trade for some fresh produce? I know a woman who used to babysit a neighbours' child once a week in exchange for a basket of vegetables.

Local Farmers' Markets are a wonderful option for fresh produce as it is usually fresher and more nutritious than food shipped across the globe. If you cannot afford it, many jurisdictions provide food stamps or coupons to use at local farmers' markets. For example, in British Columbia, the *Farmers' Market Nutrition Coupon Program* provides pre-paid coupons for low-income individuals to purchase fresh produce each week. Look online to see if there is a program in your city that you can take advantage of.

While we are on the subject of food assistance, if you receive a food bank donation box, the food is often high in carbohydrates and sugar. I remember looking at one basket and there were several boxes of Kraft Dinner, a giant container of candy, three cans of tomato soup, a box of white rice, meat that had already expired and a few horribly bruised apples. Now, I am not trying to say anything negative about those wonderful people who work at the food bank or those who donate to this worthy cause. The fact is that pasta, cereal, rice and canned food are the most common donated foods due to spoilage.

One way to make these foods healthier is to toss the candy (because no one needs it) and add fresh or frozen vegetables to the pasta or rice. Mix brown rice with the white rice, and a low sugar cereal with the boxed cereal to make them go further. If the food is spoiled, take it back as they may exchange it for another product. Some places have an option to obtain fresh produce while others do not. Using as much of the food provided allows you to use your money to purchase healthy options that are not included.

Recipe: Snack Box Lunch

Ingredients:

1 bell pepper sliced (choose their favourite kind)
¼ cucumber (sliced)
1 apple (sliced) or grapes
3 pieces deli turkey (rolled into tube)
Cheese cubes or cheese stick
edamame
Hummus dip
6 whole grain crackers
1 hard boiled egg
¼ cup mixed nuts and seeds (caution: peanuts are often forbidden at school)

Purchase a snack box or multiple small containers and add in a variety of vegetables, cut up fruit, hummus dip or natural nut butter such as almond butter or peanut butter (if the school allows it), rolled deli meats and whole grain crackers.

Add this mixture in a thermos of cold unsweetened tea or water bottle and you have a great meal they will enjoy.

Chapter Seventeen: Is Organic Really Necessary?

"Came from a plant, eat it
Made in a plant, don't."
-Michael Pollen

17

I have often been asked if organic food is necessary. After all, it is more expensive than other fruits and vegetables. When you are on a budget, buying organic food seems like a luxury and maybe not worth the while.

The argument for organic food stems from two main areas: genetically modified (GM) or genetically engineered (GE) foods and chemicals (herbicides and pesticides) that are sprayed on the plants and in the ground, which are deemed a risk to our health and environment.

A GM is a seed, plant, animal, or fish that has been genetically modified in a laboratory using genetic engineering. This could result in a product that is a combination of plant, animal, bacteria, and virus genes that does not occur naturally in nature or through traditional cross breeding methods. While the government has deemed GM seeds safe for human consumption, opposition groups believe the risk is too high for our health and the environment. Many of these products have been banned in some European countries, as the risks have been deemed too high, but are still used in North America.

It is important to remember that humans have been selectively crossbreeding animals and plants for generations to produce a more desired trait. Whether this is a flower with a greater scent or different color, or a dog that doesn't shed, or a cow that is able to withstand colder winters, selective breeding is the method used. The problem is that there may be unwanted traits, mixed results and selective breeding can take a longer time.

Scientists argue that by using modern genetic bioengineering, the problems with traditional selective breeding are eliminated.

Genetically engineered animals have been on the market for years, such as chickens with enlarged breasts, or salmon that have been created to mature faster for consumption at eighteen months instead of three years when they would be naturally grown to maturity. When we purchase these products at the grocery store, we may not be aware that these are GM products.

A GM seed or plant could be modified to improve the nutritional value of the product, resist insects or change the product itself. They are created to provide a benefit for the consumer. For example, seedless watermelon or grapes are very convenient when feeding your toddler (because picking out those seeds is a pain in the butt). In Hawaii, the papaya industry was plagued by ring spot virus which no traditional or organic farming methods was able to eliminate. Now, with genetically modified papaya that is resistant to the virus, the industry in Hawaii was saved.

When farmers grow one crop (called a mono crop) and the plants die due to insect infestation, the entire crop is lost, and the food will not be available for market. The companies that produce the GM seeds, herbicides and pesticides argue that these seeds ensure higher yielding crops, and more production means we can feed more people.

Organic farmers argue that eliminating mono crops and having a diverse growing field (with a variety of vegetables, fruits or grains) allows nature to ensure food is available for market. This was the type of garden grown by our grandparents, which you may be familiar with. When a plant has to survive insects, it becomes stronger and more naturally resilient. An insect may eat one particular type of plant, but the rest of the field will be untouched. Insects that destroy plants also have beneficial insects that feed on them, creating a balanced ecology. Organic practices are not harmful to bees, birds, native plant life or waterways. Diverse farming is a more traditional farming, and has been shown to produce just as much, if not more, food for the market.

Some GM seeds are genetically modified with glyphosate herbicide (round up) chemicals to prevent insects from destroying the plant and therefore ensuring a better crop for the farmer. But the question is, if the plant contains the chemical, and we eat the plant, aren't we eating the same chemical? How is this healthy for us? Common crops that contain this type of GM seed are wheat, alfalfa, soybeans, sugar beets, corn, and canola. Approximately 75% of these crops end up in processed foods and are used in feeding cows and chickens raised for slaughter.

According to the Food and Drug Administration, foods that are genetically modified with glyphosate are 'safe for human consumption.' Now, I am not a scientist, but if it has been proven that a chemical is carcinogenic and increases the risk of cancer, and the bottle of round up tells me not to ingest it, then why is it safe to genetically add this to our food?

A recent issue that has surfaced is that of insects evolving to combat the 'roundup ready crop,' creating new 'super bugs' and weeds evolving to become herbicide resistant. This means that stronger chemicals must be used to provide the same level of production.

As assessment of the environmental impact of the high use of herbicides, pesticides, chemical fertilizers and GM seeds has shown negative impact on our water, air, soil and native plants.

Pesticides are classified as possible carcinogenic (or carcinogenic depending on which report you read) to humans and may cause asthma, cancer, respiratory illness, ADHD, muscle weakness and skin rash. As a greater number of pesticides are used, these products are spread into the air, water and our food sources.

Effects of herbicide exposure ranges from vomiting, nausea, and skin rashes to death, depending on the product used. These products also leach into the water and are spread into the air by wind and rainfall. The exposure of these chemicals is not limited to the immediate area surrounding the farm; even polar bears have been found to have toxic chemicals.

There is also the controversy of whether organic food is more nutritious and depending on which study you read, you will get a different answer. I believe if you use a chemical fertilizer, the roots of the plant are absorbing that chemical inside the cell walls. Ultimately, when we ingest the plant, we ingest the chemical. Scientists state that these chemicals do not reduce the nutrition of the food while environmental groups say they do.

Studies funded by chemical companies will show that the GM seeds are safe for human consumption and produce better results for the market. Studies funded by non-GM companies, organic food groups or environmental groups will show that GM seeds have a higher risk for health, higher risk for environmental impact and no real benefit for the consumer.

There are studies that have shown that GM foods are creating issues of allergies (because one plant is being crossed with another), toxicity, auto-immune disorders, cancer, antibiotic resistance and a loss of nutrition. According to the *Environmental Working Group*, glyphosate (the chemical in round up) doubles the risk of blood cancer and in a report released by the International Agency for Research on Cancer, it stated that glyphosate is carcinogenic to animals in laboratory studies. The results from the NutriNet-Sante Prospective Cohort study indicate a twenty-five percent reduced risk of cancer, especially breast and prostate cancer, for those who ate organic foods rather than non-organic foods.

Because GM foods are relatively new, there isn't a lot of information about the long-term health effects of consuming these products. Whether for the lack of long-term studies, religious reasons or a belief that Mother Nature isn't to be tampered with; many people are choosing to avoid GM foods and eat organic foods instead.

To be honest, unless you are extremely rigorous, or only eat food you grow yourself, you will still be ingesting some GM foods. There are so many on the market that you probably won't be able to avoid all of them, but you can choose to reduce your consumption by eating organic foods.

Requirements for organic food labels vary from country to country. In Canada, a 'Certified Organic' label is only displayed on products that are made of ninety-five percent organic ingredients and must contain the name of the certifying organization. Terms such as 'grown organically' or 'organic produce' follow the same rules. Canada does not allow the use of 'made with organic ingredients' because it isn't clear how much of the product is truly organic. Here in Canada, there is a logo attached to all organic products, which makes it much easier for us to identify.

The United States has similar requirements for the label of 'organic' on their products. They allow '100% organic' if the product is one hundred percent organic and 'Organic' if it contains a minimum of 95%. 'Made with organic___' is allowed if the product has at least 70% organically produced ingredients. There are also several logos that allow consumers to identify organic products more easily.

If you want to reduce your risk of pesticides from non-organic foods, try running them under clean water for twenty minutes. Scrub the outside of the fruit or vegetable with a vegetable scrubber or peel off the skin. This may help to reduce the risk of any residual pesticides that are on the surface of the food, however, you are also losing the nutrients contained in the skin. You can also soak them in a vinegar and water mixture for twenty minutes to help wash off any residue.

If you want to eat organic but cannot afford to have all organic food, the Environmental Working Group produces a list of the *dirty dozen,* or the foods with the highest amount of pesticide residue. Currently the list includes:

- Strawberries
- Spinach
- Kale, Collard, and Mustard Greens
- Peaches
- Pears
- Nectarines
- Apples
- Grapes
- Bell and Hot Peppers
- Cherries
- Blueberries
- Green beans

If you choose to eat organic, the *dirty dozen* are the foods that I would focus on first. By eliminating or reducing your processed foods, you will automatically be reducing your intake of the GM crops mentioned earlier in this chapter. Organic hormone free meats are also available at grocery stores, butcher shops or specialty shops.

You can also find organic foods at your local farmer's market. Just be sure to ask them about their pesticide and herbicide practices and whether they use traditional non-genetically modified seeds for their plants. This way, you can be certain that they are truly organic. Grocery stores are now selling more organic produce at a much lower cost than ever before, and even *Amazon Fresh* has a large selection of organic foods if you choose to shop online.

Eating organic doesn't have to be super expensive or complicated if you don't want it to be. I tell my clients to use their common sense and do what feels right to them. There will be times when they eat organic healthy foods and times when they will eat whatever is available to them. They may choose to grow their own food or feel that the risk of GM products is not a concern to them.

Recipe: Spaghetti Squash Spaghetti

Ingredients

1 spaghetti squash
1 pkg (approx. 1 lb) lean ground turkey or chicken
1 can no salt tomato sauce
1 can diced tomatoes
½ onion diced
3 cloves garlic minced
1 bell pepper diced
3 mushrooms diced
Extra virgin olive oil
1 tbsp. Italian seasoning
Optional: ½ cup shredded cheese (mozzarella or parmesan)

Cut off the ends of the squash, then slice lengthwise and remove seeds.
Place face down in baking dish with ½ cup water and cover with tinfoil.
Bake at 350 degrees for 45 to 60 minutes (depending on size of squash). When you can easily prick the skin with a fork, it means that it is done.

Put olive oil in frying pan and cook meat over medium high temperature until cooked thoroughly. Break apart with wooden spoon while cooking.

Add in vegetables and cook approximately 4 minutes.

Lower temperature to medium-low, add in tomato sauce, diced tomatoes and seasoning. Simmer until all vegetables are cooked, and squash is ready.

Carefully remove squash from oven. Turn over squash and use fork in a scraping motion to remove the flesh. It will look like spaghetti. Place in a bowl.

Add squash to individual bowls, top with meat sauce and shredded cheese and serve immediately or place squash in casserole dish and top with meat sauce and cheese and bake for 15 minutes longer for drier squash.

Chapter Eighteen: Change isn't Easy

"The secret of change is to focus all of your energy, not on fighting the old, but on building the new."

-Socrates

18

Effective dietary changes with your child will greatly depend on their age and 'buy-in' for the changes. Making changes for a small child when you control all of the purchasing and providing of food is easier than with a teenager who will go elsewhere for the food they desire.

Imagine for a moment you have decided to go on a diet and are not going to eat any of your favourite sugary sweet foods. You get a craving, but you are able to motivate yourself to restrict your eating because you have chosen this diet. Now imagine your spouse has decided you are at an unhealthy weight, and they are restricting your favourite foods, but you get a food craving. Let's say you really want a brownie, and your spouse tells you no, because it is not part of the diet they have set for you. How happy are you going to be with your spouse? Are you going to smile and say 'Oh thanks dear! I know you have my best interests at heart'? No! You are going to argue, yell, call them names, and go out and buy your brownie. This is the same attitude you may deal with as you put your older child 'on a diet' without buy-in.

If you think of this as a healthy eating plan for life, it does not feel restrictive and allows for the occasional unhealthy food. If you are very strict with a child, you will have issues. So, unless the child has developed diabetes and therefore their diet must be more restrictive, I am going to recommend a more gradual balanced approach. This will prevent as many cravings as possible, temper tantrums and fights in the home.

Depending on the age of your child, changing their diet can be a bit tricky, so start by doing an assessment of what your child eats and drinks in a day when they are with you, at school, or out with friends. How many sugary drinks are they consuming? What are they snacks they like eating? How much processed foods are they consuming? What are their portion sizes? Do they eat after-dinner right before bed? Are they hanging around with people who eat larger meals or are more sedentary?

Once you have made an assessment, make changes gradually! Start small and continue to make healthier choices as you go. Decide where you want to start. Maybe it will be breakfast? Buy a healthier version of cereal or oatmeal instead of pop tarts. Switch from white bread to whole grain. Buy natural peanut butter instead of the one that contains molasses, sugar, salt, preservatives, and other fillers. Maybe it will be dinner when the whole family is together, and you can provide a healthier meal?

My mother taught me to pick my battles in order to win the war; and you will not win the war when you are waging it on all fronts. As the parent, you must decide what changes you want to start with, because changing everything at once will not work and will stress you out. If your child is old enough and is eager to change their diet and lifestyle, then perhaps, deciding together which changes you will start with would be the best option. Remember, the changes you are making will be for the entire family, so choose to start where you are comfortable as well.

A client decided to start with sugary drinks as her son was addicted to soda, Gatorade and Kool-Aid, and she estimated he drank over 2,000 extra calories per day from this addiction. She bought him a really nice water bottle and stickers to decorate it to try and entice him to drink more water. Then she stopped buying soda except for one small bottle on Saturday night for family movie night. She reduced the amount of sugar in the Kool-Aid gradually. Then she stopped buying Kool-Aid altogether and told him to drink water or milk.

I would love to say this was an easy transition and that her son was happy throughout the changes, but that would be a lie. He screamed, yelled, threw things, called his mother names and was a holy terror. When they were at the store, he would constantly ask for soda and even fight with her to put it in the grocery cart, so she stopped taking him to the store. He would go to his friend's house and ask for soda but because his mother spoke with the other parents, they refused him. He even snuck out to the store and bought some himself. It was a very challenging time for the family. Sugar addiction affects the same parts of the brain as cocaine or other drugs, so the withdrawal and cravings can be fierce. After a few weeks, it became less and less of an issue until even the Saturday night soda was stopped. His mother stayed strong because she knew his health was at stake, but it was not easy for her.

Another common issue is the 'once in a while' slippery slope. Imagine you are out with your family, it has been a long day, and you are too tired to cook, so you stop by the grocery store or fast-food place to pick up something quick. Someone suggests a piece of cake and you agree. Then a week later the same thing happens, but you tell yourself that it is okay and 'once in a while' will not hurt. However, the problem is that you need to define 'once in a while' or it becomes a regular occurrence. As humans, we are creatures of habit, so we will slip back into old unhealthy habits. I am not telling you to never eat cake or go to a fast-food restaurant again, but I am telling you to define how often, which ones, and what you will order. Telling yourself you will never have a specific food item that you love will make you want it more.

You may find that posting your weekly menu where everyone can see may help keep the meals on track. If you don't follow the menu and instead eat processed food or take-out food, then mark the date in red ink to make it stand out. At a glance, you will be able to see if you are keeping to your plan, and this also allows you to ensure you are eating enough vegetables, lean proteins and whole natural grains and not slip back into old cooking and eating habits.

One of the biggest challenges you will face is changing your own habits and making the extra effort (on top of everything else you have going on) to change the habits of your child. They are watching what you say and do. When my daughter was a toddler and learning to speak, we did not realize how much she was really paying attention to everything going on around her. One day we were sitting at the back of the church and the minister called out 'God' to which my daughter yelled back at the top of her lungs 'Dammit!' and every eye in the church turned to look at us. Do not believe for a second your child is not watching and hearing everything you do and say.

As a parent, you need to set the example for your child; if you are eating and drinking unhealthy food on a regular basis, then so will your child. If you are constantly eating on the run from take-out restaurants, then so will they. If you are using slim fast, or lean cuisine meals, then so will they. If the parent is eating healthy and exercising, the child is more likely to follow suit. Remember, they want to be like you, and as the adult, you must lead by example.

I want to talk about the language you use for yourself. If you are constantly talking about your latest diet, or that you are fat or hate your body, then the child will adopt the same attitude. If you say things such as 'I am going to be bad and have a cookie' then you are equating food with poor behaviour. If you are constantly looking in the mirror and saying you need to lose ten pounds to be attractive, then your child will hear the same message.

We have far more influence on our young children than we realize; when you are talking about your own eating habits, use the same words you would for your child. Talk about exercising for strength and agility, and about eating for stronger bones or muscles. Use words of love and acceptance to describe your body rather than talking about having to lose five pounds so you look good in a bathing suit or fit into a specific size of clothing. Language matters, and they are listening.

Talk with your child about their weight and encourage them to share their feelings and thoughts. Make sure you are actively listening; and if you have had similar experiences, it might help to share them. Reassure them you love them no matter what size they are, and always will. Use language such as 'we are going to get healthier as a family' not 'you are on a diet.' Describe foods as healthy, or this food gives us strong bones, or this food gives us good eyesight. Do not describe food as 'bad' or 'fattening' as this may create an unhealthy relationship with food. Children tend to equate behaviors with self-esteem; for example, because they eat 'bad' food they are bad. Or because they eat 'fattening' food they are fat. You get the idea. Language is important!

It is up to you to be the role model for healthy behaviour, to purchase natural whole foods and reduce the processed sugary foods in the house, and to suggest going to the park, or for a walk, or to play ball. I would love to tell you that changing their food will help them lose weight and get healthy, but the truth is that a healthy lifestyle is a combination of food, exercise, sleep habits and stress management. This change is going to require continuous effort on your part.

Being a parent is a full-time forever job but the most important one in the world. It may sound like I am putting all of the onus on you and for the most part I am. In my experience, because the parent runs the house, you will need to make the necessary adjustments before anything changes. Older children have a part to play, but ultimately, they will look to you for guidance.

While you are making changes, remember that it is not enough to change the diet and lifestyle of one child in your home; this is a lifestyle change for the whole family. We don't want to single out one member, making them feel responsible for the other members of the family. For example, if you do not allow ice cream into the house because one child is prediabetic or overweight, the other child may make comments about the lack of ice cream, making the unhealthy child feel responsible or unhappy, and the healthy child resentful of the other. You need to adopt a healthy diet and lifestyle that the whole family can live with, food and activities that all of you enjoy and a lifestyle you can live with. This is not a diet – this is a lifestyle.

While the majority of the time, the food in the household needs to be healthy, allow the occasional treat on your monthly 'free day' to accommodate all members of the home. If your child is insulin dependent, the 'treat' may need to be discussed with their doctor in order to keep their blood sugar balanced but remember to make this a rare occasion. Most of the diet needs to be based on healthy, natural foods without added sugars or anything highly processed.

I encourage you to reward your child with something other than food for good behaviour. I'm sure that every parent has told their child if they behaved at the dentist or are brave while getting vaccinations, then you will take them to get a treat (I know I have) because bribery is a reality in parenting. Instead of using food, think of other rewards such as a new toy, or a fun activity or just words of praise that may motivate your child. I know this can be a creative challenge for the parents, but we need to stop using food as a bribe or reward. Food is just nutrition and other than very special occasions such as a birthday, it should not be anything but what we consume every day for our health.

Most parents that I know are stressed out, burned-out and often exhausted. They work full time and sometimes have a side hustle to make ends meet, are responsible for the cooking and cleaning and are the primary caregiver for the children. These parents have a lot going on and don't need to be told to add another thing to their plate or that they aren't doing a good job. It is not my intention to tell a parent that they need to do better, but I am saying you may need to do it differently.

The suggestions that I make are all about changing the way you do things, and not trying to add more onto your plate. Remember that you don't have to be a Superhero, and leaning on your spouse, family, friends, or community is perfectly acceptable. Maybe you have a family member or friend who can take your child out to the park while you have some down time? Maybe you can get a friend to watch your child while you go grocery shopping and then you return the favour? Try to think of ways that you can lean on the people in your life to make healthy changes without causing unnecessary stress for you. I know you are a strong and amazing parent and will figure out how to make the best changes for your child.

In the end, it all comes down to you. I know you are super busy. Finding the time to follow these suggestions can seem impossible but remember you don't have to do everything. Start small and gradually make bigger changes. Do what feels right to you for your family. You will have good days, and you will have bad days but when you became a parent, you were given the superpowers of love and persistence and I know you have the strength to make this happen.

Recipe: Blueberry Chia Pancakes

No need for syrup as these pancakes are already sweet.

Ingredients:

1 cup quick cooking oats
½ cup oat milk (plain unsweetened) or cow's milk
1 banana medium size
1 egg large
1 tsp baking powder
1 cup frozen blueberries
1 ½ tsp chia seeds
1 tbsp extra virgin olive oil

Add oats to a blender and blend to a flour consistency (about 30 seconds) then add milk, banana, egg, and baking powder. Blend until smooth scraping down the sides as needed. Gently stir in blueberries and chia seeds.

Heat the oil in a non-stick pan over medium heat. Pour ¼ cup of batter at a time and cook 2-3 minutes per side until cooked through.

Serve immediately.

Chapter Nineteen: Collaborating with your Doctor

"Family is not an important thing. It's everything."

-Michael J. Fox

19

Discussing your child's weight with your doctor may be an embarrassing subject, or maybe you just assume your doctor will tell you if they think there is a problem, however, many doctors will not speak up unless you say something first. If you think there may be a problem, ask your doctor if your child's weight is within normal range for a child their age. They will calculate their body mass index to determine if it is within a normal percentile. If your child is overweight, they may offer suggestions such as changing their diet, more exercise or lifestyle changes.

Some questions that you may choose to ask your physician are:
- What is their goal weight range?
- What activities can we do as a family to help them get better health?
- How can I help them develop better eating habits?
- Are there any resources in my community that can assist me?
- How can I get my child to choose healthy foods without nagging at them?
- Should I talk to them about the food commercials we see on TV? What should I say?
- How will puberty affect their weight?
- How can I motivate them without them feeling badly about themselves?
- My teenager always seems hungry. Is this normal?
- How much taller will they grow? Will they grow into their weight?

- The other parent allows them to eat whatever they want. How should I deal with this?
- I think my child has an eating disorder. What should I do?

If the weight gain continues, or the child shows signs of illness, your doctor may run a series of tests to determine if they are becoming insulin resistant or type 2 diabetic. Depending on your child's medical situation, your doctors may prescribe metformin or similar drugs to help reduce weight, while other doctors realize the long-term negative effect of these medications and instead choose to work with the family to create a healthier lifestyle to naturally reverse this syndrome. If you are uncomfortable with your doctor's recommendations, you are entitled to a second opinion. As a mother, I believe in listening to my instincts about the health of my child, and they haven't let me down yet.

Always work with your doctor and do not restrict the calories of a child without consulting their doctor first. Children are still growing and have certain caloric needs depending on their age and growth cycle. It is quite common for physicians to keep them at their current caloric intake and allow them to 'grow into' the caloric range rather than limiting calories.

You can also work with a nutritionist like myself, to visit the home and work with the whole family to create healthier eating habits. We explain healthy foods versus unhealthy foods, food swaps, give ideas that are focused on problem areas or suggest changes that may be of benefit. Sometimes we will teach the children to make a fun and delicious snack as part of the training, which I have found most kids love to do.

If you are worried your child has an eating disorder or unhealthy relationship with food, please get them the professional help they need. Speak to your doctor for a referral and support them while they work through this issue. Eating disorders, chronic dieting, and starvation diets take a terrible toll on the physical and mental health of a child and early intervention is key.

Signs to look out for include refusing to eat, excusing themselves after a meal and vomiting, hiding food in their room, binge eating, using laxatives, disruptions in normal eating patterns, being unusually preoccupied with their body image, dizziness, fainting, refusing to eat around other people, or extreme weight loss.

Time for some more hard truth here. If you have an eating disorder or unhealthy relationship with food, your child is more likely to have one too. Parents model eating behaviours and relationship to food. Mothers who talk more frequently about their own weight, shape or size are more likely to have daughters with a lower feeling of self-worth because the child will model themselves after the parent. Eating disorders run in families and fifty to eighty percent of children with an eating disorder have a parent with one as well.

Now, I am not telling you this to blame or shame anyone, but I want you to become more aware of the risks associated with eating disorders, constant dieting and body hating. If you are a parent with body dysmorphia, an eating disorder, a bad relationship with food (you see food as the enemy) or openly talk about hating your body – please get the help you need. You cannot tell your child one thing and then do the opposite, because it doesn't work. Your whole family deserves to be happy and healthy, and that includes you.

Recipe: Vegetarian Chilli

Ingredients:

2 large can (28 oz) kidney beans or 3 small (15 oz)
cans, rinsed and drained.
1 can (15 oz) black beans rinsed and drained.
1 large can (28oz) diced tomatoes
1 can low sodium tomato sauce
2 tbsp extra virgin olive oil
1 medium onion chopped (white or red)
1 large red bell pepper chopped
3 medium carrots peeled and diced
3 sticks of celery chopped
4 cloves garlic minced
2 tbsp chilli powder
2 tsp ground cumin
1 tsp dried oregano
1 tsp paprika (optional: adds spicy flavor)
1 cup low sodium vegetable broth or water
Chopped cilantro

If you are using a slow cooker, add all ingredients, stir and cook on low during the day. Or in large pot, add oil over medium heat, add onion, bell pepper, carrot and celery. Cook approximately 7 minutes stirring frequently.

Add in garlic and spices, cook for 1 minute.

Add in tomato sauce, diced tomatoes, beans, and broth or water. Stir and bring to a simmer reducing heat as needed. Cook 30 minutes.

Serve in individual bowls with cilantro garnish.

Chapter Twenty: Emotional Support

"No one would feel embarrassed about seeking help for a child if they broke their arm – and we really should be equally ready to support a child coping with emotional difficulties."

-Kate Middleton

20

Sometimes as parents, we are so busy with the physical needs of parenting (making food, doing laundry, buying groceries, washing dishes) that we forget about the emotional needs that also require attention. Children need unconditional love, encouragement, validation, boundaries, a sense of control and to feel as though they are important; and if they aren't getting this from their parents, they will seek it out elsewhere.

Food can serve as a replacement to meet an emotional need for a child (or an adult). This is because certain foods produce endorphins (the feel-good emotion), which can be part of a soothing behaviour when a child does not have their emotional needs met. For example, if the parents are fighting, the child may eat to feel better because they are anxious or sad. Common triggers for emotional eating are sadness, anxiety, stress, boredom, feeling of emptiness, exerting control over the body or environment, or social influence.

As children, we also learn emotional eating behaviours from our parents. If we received a food as compensation for a job well done, such as a Dairy Queen Blizzard for a good report card, then we will associate this food as a celebratory food and crave it when we have a success in our life. If our parents gave us food when we cried, then we will crave food to fulfill that emotional need. The problem with emotional eating is that after the food is gone, the emotion is still there and needs to be addressed.

As a society, we need to learn to stop using food for comfort and understand that its purpose is to supply us with nutrition. You can train your young children to use non-food mechanisms such as thinking happy thoughts, distraction, getting hugs from loved one or affection from a pet to create the dopamine needed to feel better; this will help during difficult times. As parents, we need to stop offering food as a prize (such as for good grades) or for comfort (such as after the dentist or when they are sad).

Teenagers that are accustomed to using food for comfort will need more help, as their habits are more ingrained. Offer a glass of water or cup of tea and sit and listen to them talk about their problems. Don't try to solve them, just listen without judgement. If they want your advice, they will let you know. Some teens will need more help than you can give them, such as a counsellor or therapist. Not dealing with negative emotions can trigger different eating disorders such as binge eating, anorexia or bulimia. If you need help finding a counselor for your teen; talk to their doctor, school or minister for referrals.

Have you ever pulled on your favourite pants only to find they are too snug and no longer look good on you? You need to be out the door in twenty minutes and have nothing that fits? Now add adolescent hormones, peer pressure and anxiety and you understand some of what your teenager is going through. Clothes that don't fit or look good, bullying, not feeling attractive, not having friends, not having the energy to keep trying when nothing is working – this is a typical day in the life of a child with weight issues. There are a lot of emotions going on and it is important that our children learn to address the emotions through actions such as talking, writing, deep breathing or exercise and not food.

As a parent, we want to make things better. We want to fix things because we think that is our job. Ever since our child was little, we were there to kiss the boo-boos and make the boogeyman disappear. It is in our nature to want to do something, to take action, to find a solution. Sadly, there are times when our parent superpowers don't work and all we can do is be there in a supportive role. For me, this is extremely difficult as I am a problem solver. It's what I do for a living in my nutrition practice, it's what I do at home and not being able to fix the problem is agonizing.

One thing I learned the hard way is that sometimes my daughter didn't want me to solve the problem, but just to listen to her. To be there for her without doing anything or making suggestions. To give her a hug and tell her she is beautiful, smart, and funny. To make her feel wanted and loved. This was my most important job and to be honest, sometimes I failed.

Ways that you can support your child include:

- Listening to them without judgement or blame.
- Offering them encouragement.
- Being patient when they are having a melt down.
- Let your child be a part of the solution and learn to take control of the situation.
- Talk about the things they do well. Boost self-esteem by focusing on what a unique individual they are. Maybe they are creative, kind, smart or talented?
- Focus on health not weight.

- Tell them they are beautiful/handsome, and you love them no matter what size they are.
- Don't trivialize their concerns or how they are feeling.
- Spend quality time with them without distractions and let them know they are a priority.
- If they won't talk to you, find someone they trust to open up about their challenges and concerns.
- If you have similar experiences, talk about how you felt and how you can sympathize with them.

Feeling heard provides a feeling of validation and respect in kids, and this supports their self-esteem and helps them to be more receptive to listening to what we have to say. With teenagers, this may mean acknowledging what they are saying even if we disagree with them and letting them voice their frustrations without responding to the way they voice them. We still need to teach them to express their feelings respectfully and without violence but if they need to raise their voice or cry or even swear, sometimes it is better just to be silent and supportive and help them get it out.

One of the most important ways that we can support and influence the behaviour of our kids is by spending quality time with them. The truth is that the impact of spending time will influence your child for the rest of their life more than any other activity.

Let me give you an example. Ask any adult about the toys their parents bought for them over their lifetime, and they might remember one or two, but ask them about memories of their parents or the top ten memories they have of their parents, and they will remember time spent doing something with them.

My greatest memories of my mom are not the toys she bought me, or a computer game, but spending time with her in dusty second-hand bookstores on a treasure hunt for a specific book or sitting at the kitchen table doing a puzzle with her talking about things going on in my life at the time. It was when she volunteered with my Brownie troop and took me door to door selling cookies in the pouring rain holding an umbrella over me, so my box of cookies didn't get wet, or cheered me on at my soccer games, even though she hated sports. It was the time spent with her that impacted and influenced me the most and shaped me into the woman I am today. If we want to have more influence over our kids and support them, then spending quality time with them is key.

I know that time is the one thing we all wish we had more of, yet it seems to pass so quickly. We never seem to have enough time to do everything we want and need to do. Time can be our enemy or friend, but we can make the time we spend with our children be more effective by becoming aware of our actions.

I watched a woman and her daughter the other day at the park. The little girl was playing on the slide and the mom was on her cell phone texting and ignoring her daughter. The little girl kept asking her mom to play but the mom was too busy on her phone to notice. Then the mother started taking selfies and asked the little girl to smile and pose with her, which she did. After returning to her phone again (assumedly to send the new selfies), the mom announced it was time to go and started packing up to leave. She never played with the girl or spent any quality time with her. The memory that will be left with this little girl will be of her mom being more interested in her phone and sending selfies than playing with her and making her feel unimportant. Although she was technically spending time with her daughter, she wasn't spending quality time.

Without adding anymore to your already busy plate, take note of the time you spend with your child. Perhaps a few adjustments to the time you are already spending can provide you better results. Think about your day-to-day activities with your child/children. Are you actively speaking with them or are you ignoring them in favour of your cell phone or the television? How much quality time are you spending together? If you feel that you need to spend more time with them, why not do something active together? Read a book to your little one or play basketball with your teenager or go for a walk or any activity that gets you talking together. I'm not telling you to spend every waking moment with your child but try and create some dedicated time together and ensure that you are positively influencing their behaviour and making them feel important in your life.

I realize that I have suggested you add more into your busy schedule and if you are anything like me, you probably already have a very full plate. As parents we often feel stretched too thin which is why it is important to also take care of your own emotional health. Don't be afraid to ask for help when you need it and take some time for yourself. When my daughter was little, I got seriously burned out and to cope, I started having what I called my '*me day*' once a month. Truthfully, this day was only a couple of hours to have peace and quiet, to go shopping for myself or get my hair cut or have a bath without anyone banging on the door; but this precious time saved my sanity.

I believe that, as parents, we need to recharge our batteries to stay happier, healthier, which allows us to continuously give our best. We work at jobs outside the home, we are responsible for the shopping, food preparation, house cleaning, laundry, child rearing and a list a mile long of things we need to get done. Taking a little time for yourself is essential not selfish, so be sure to schedule this time off. Maybe you can get your spouse to take over for this period or another family member? Or trade days with a friend so each of you can get some time off? Make this me day a priority in your life and don't give it up too easily. Treat it like an appointment you must keep, and if your spouse or boss asks you to give up this day, make sure it is for a really good reason and then reschedule it or you will find this time gets stolen away because it is not a priority in someone else's life.

Recipe: No-Bake Protein Balls

Ingredients:

1 cup nut or seed butter of choice (peanut butter, sunflower, almond butter)

5 pitted dates

¼ cup protein powder (organic plain or vanilla sweetened with stevia)

¾ cup hemp seeds

¼ cup chia seeds

Place all ingredients in a food processor and blend until combined.

Roll into balls using 1 tbsp of mixture.

Place on parchment paper and pop into fridge for 15 minutes. Keep refrigerated.

Tip:

Roll the balls into unsweetened shredded coconut, cacao powder or sesame seeds for a fun taste.

Chapter Twenty-One: Are they Getting Enough Sleep?

"Without enough sleep, we all become tall two year olds."
-JoJo Jensen

21

According to the Center for Disease Control, there are three main contributors to weight gain in children, and a lack of quality sleep is one of them. Sleep deprivation can lead to hormonal imbalances, which causes food cravings, especially for foods high in sugar to provide instant energy. Sleep deprivation can also impact our healing and growing. A study at Emory University in Atlanta showed that not only do growth spurts happen during sleep, but longer, deeper sleep can affect body length during our growing years.

Preschoolers need ten to thirteen hours of sleep (including naps) and researchers have found that preschoolers that go to bed before 8pm cut their risk of obesity in half. School aged children (6 to 12 years of age) require nine to twelve hours of sleep and teenagers (13 to 18 years of age) need eight to ten hours of sleep a night.

Sleep is an essential function for our body that allows our brain to remove toxins, recharge, helps our body to heal, causes growth hormone to be released, helps muscles to grow, and increases energy and cognitive abilities. If you have ever been sleep deprived, then you would know how difficult it can be to think, function, and have adequate control of emotions (remember how you felt when your baby wasn't sleeping through the night?) and because children are growing, it is critical for them to get adequate sleep every night. You are not being mean by insisting on a regular bedtime even on weekends; you are taking care of their physical, mental, and emotional health. Remember, you are their parent not their friend, so it is your job to set healthy rules and boundaries even if your child doesn't like it.

Improve your child's quality of sleep by ensuring a regular bedtime that allows them to have eight to ten hours of sleep per night including on weekends. Stop all electronics at least an hour before bedtime; shut off any electronics in their room to stop any blue light (this interferes with REM sleep) and make the room dark and quiet. If you live in a noisy neighborhood, try playing white noise in the background by using a fan or humidifier. Remove pets from the bedroom (especially those that are active at night), as children are more susceptible to pet dander and allergies.

Over time, fungi, bacteria, dust mites and dander can cluster in the pillow, which can create breathing issues, allergies, and illness such as lung infections and in rare cases even death. As anyone with a head cold knows, if you are not breathing properly, then you won't sleep properly. Each night, our body sheds approximately fifteen million skin cells and one study found that pillowcases can harbour more bacteria than a toilet seat. Be sure to wash your pillowcases and sheets regularly, and your pillows every three months and change them out once per year.

Wash pillows using oxygen bleach (it will also help with the yellowing) in hot water to kill any germs. Using a mattress cover can not only protect the mattress from dirt and sweat, but also prevent dust mites and dander from collecting in the mattress. Wash your mattress cover regularly in hot water and oxygen bleach to keep it clean and smelling fresh.

Using a humidifier will increase the moisture in the air, which has been shown to improve sleep quality. Dry air makes sinuses feel tight and congested, which can disrupt sleep and cause snoring. A humidifier can also help those with respiratory issues such as asthma by keeping the airways properly lubricated, which allows the phlegm to flow properly, reducing the frequency of asthma attacks. In addition to helping the respiratory system, a higher rate of humidity can feel soothing to the skin, especially to those with eczema or skin allergies. If your child wakes with a stuffed-up nose, chapped lips, or dry skin, they may find a humidifier very beneficial. The white noise of the machine can also be very soothing and help block outside noises that may disrupt sleep. Be sure to clean the humidifier regularly according to the manufacturer's instructions or you can end up with mildew in the machine, which can make you sick.

Researchers have shown that children with a shorter sleep duration have higher insulin levels, more insulin sensitivity (their body does not process insulin and glucose correctly), which leads to weight gain. Lack of sleep decreases our available energy; therefore, we are less physically active and have a greater desire for food (especially sugary foods) to provide us energy. A lack of sleep also creates physical and emotional stress on the body and an inability to process stressful events. It is important that your child should have a good sleep schedule and a proper night's rest.

Recipe: Mini Breakfast Quiche

Ingredients:

1 tbsp extra virgin olive oil
¼ cup onion diced (white or red)
¼ cup red bell pepper diced (really small)
2 cup baby spinach chopped
½ cup shredded cheese – Cheddar or jalapeno Monterey Jack
¼ cup milk
4 large eggs

Preheat oven to 350 degree and lightly spray 6 cup muffin tin with cooking spray.

Heat oil in pan over medium high heat. Add onion and pepper and cook until tender, add spinach and cook until spinach wilts.
Transfer contents to bowl and allow it to cool. Once cool add cheese.

Whisk milk with eggs, pour mixture over vegetables and stir to combine. Divide mixture in muffin tin and bake 20 minutes.

Serve immediately or let them cool, and cover with saran wrap or put in airtight container and refrigerate. To reuse, just pop them in the microwave to reheat or eat them cold.

Chapter Twenty-Two: Travelling Made Easier

"In the end, kids won't remember the fancy toy you
bought them, they will remember the time you spent
with them."

-Kevin Heath

22

I love travelling, but doing so with children can be a bit challenging. Boredom, fighting, bathroom breaks, car sickness, where and what to eat are all common issues; but one of the biggest difficulties I encounter is finding healthy food on the road.

Personally, I prefer driving with kids because flying is super stressful to me. If I am driving, I can stop as often as I need to, and if my granddaughter wants to listen to the same song fifty times, I can ignore it while others get angry. Regardless of how you choose to travel, there are ways to eat healthier, and save money at the same time.

If you are driving in the morning, have a good healthy breakfast at home or in a restaurant if you are already on the road. Ensure that breakfast has a protein, healthy fat, and carbohydrates that will keep them full for a while. Keep bottled water, fruit, and nuts/seeds in the car for easy snacks. These do not require refrigeration, so they are great to keep in the car or your bag. If you do have a cooler bag, string cheese, yogurt, and meat slices are a wonderful instant meal for your little one.

Some places to stop for healthier food during your travels are Love's Truck Stop, 7-Eleven, and grocery stores. Each of these places carry small packages of cheese, cut up vegetables, protein packs (usually cooked chicken), hard-boiled eggs, and fruit. Most Love's also have a subway inside so you can create a delicious sandwich full of vegetables. Grocery stores have healthy options in the deli departments such as pre-made salads, vegetables with dip, soups, and many have a salad bar as well. Focus on finding places in your area that serve food, either cooked or raw, in its natural healthy form. You can also look online before you travel to see what options are available along your route.

I would avoid McDonalds's and other fast-food restaurants and junk food during your travels, as the food is not healthy, and although it may fill their stomachs, it is not worth the convenience. High sugar content drinks and fatty foods can also upset little tummies in the car. Try and find a family restaurant that will have better options for you or create a picnic lunch from the grocery store and find a nice place to eat and stretch your legs.

Dinner time for us is always our last stop before the hotel for the night because by that time, we are ready to stop. We will have a healthy dinner of stir-fry vegetables with a protein, or salad, or another light healthy meal since you don't expend too much energy while driving. After dinner, find a place for your child to run, play and burn off their energy, so they will sleep well that night.

I recently took a trip over to Vancouver Island and while it is only five hours away, it seemed much longer with a two-year-old. We packed her formula, cheese strings, and fruit packets in the cooler box and brought her water bottle. While on the ferry, we were limited to an option of five different types of burgers, three salads with nuts (not an option because she has a nut allergy and children that young aren't crazy about lettuce) or chicken strips. We bought the chicken then asked for a side of steamed broccoli, which wasn't on the menu, but they made it for us. Don't be afraid to ask for a healthier alternative for your child. She ended up with a well-balanced meal that she enjoyed and spent the rest of the voyage playing happily in the children's play area.

Travelling by airplanes with children is all about snacks. Be sure to pack healthy snacks that each child will like such as fruit, nuts, seeds, and cut up vegetables before you leave home. Sub-sandwiches work well for the plane along with a bottle of water, but do not pack anything that has a strong smell such as eggs, or your fellow passengers will hate you. Pack food rather than buying on the plane, as you will save money, your food will be better quality and sometimes they run out of food on the plane. This has happened to us on a couple of trips. If your child is an insulin dependent diabetic always have adequate food on the plane with you.

Before you leave on your return flight, make a quick stop at a grocery store and pick up your supplies for the plane. If you are staying in an all-inclusive hotel and do not have access to a grocery store, bring enough nuts and seeds for both flights and ask the kitchen for a few bananas, oranges, and things of that sort. It has been my experience that they are always happy to oblige.

While on the plane, drink water and not soft drinks because they are quite dehydrating. I always took children's Tylenol (in case of earaches on landing) as well as Gravol and cold medicine. You do not want to be scrambling for these while you are thirty thousand feet in the air. And one more tip, do not let your children take their shoes off because feet can swell on long trips, and they may not get their shoes back on (this happened to me), so just loosen the laces for comfort.

Bring them toys and games to play with and extra batteries if required. If they are bored, they will want to eat because there is nothing else to do on a plane. Boredom eating is a real thing and when you are stuck in the air with nowhere to go, eating, sleeping or kicking the chair in front of them become the only available options. I doubt they will sleep, and kicking the chair is a bad option, which leaves eating. By bringing healthy snacks and activities for your kids, you will not only be saving money but reducing your stress as well.

Recipe: Garlic Parmesan Popcorn

Ingredients:

Plain Popcorn (air popped)
1 tbsp ground parmesan cheese (canned)
¾ tablespoon garlic powder
½ tsp dried parsley
1/8 tsp salt (optional)
½ tbsp extra virgin olive oil (amount depends on quantity of popcorn)

Mix parmesan cheese, garlic powder, parsley and salt in a small bowl.

Pop plain popcorn and while hot drizzle the olive oil over the popcorn (just enough to cover without it becoming soggy) and mix.

Sprinkle the seasoning over the popcorn and mix.

Serve immediately.

Tip:

This is a delicious snack for family movie night.

Keep leftovers in an airtight bag.

Replace olive oil with ¼ cup unsalted butter but do not keep leftovers for more than a day as butter can go rancid.

Chapter Twenty-Three: A Final Word

"It is often the small steps, not the giant leaps, that
bring about the most lasting change."

-HRM Queen Elizabeth II

23

Choosing to change your diet and lifestyle is a challenge, and it can be a bit scary or overwhelming, but I know you are making the right decision for your family. Don't be afraid to reach out for help from your doctor, a nutritionist like myself, a school counselor, local support group or spiritual leader. Raising kids is the most rewarding but hardest job in the world, and no one said you had to do it all alone.

By teaching our children to eat natural whole foods given to us by Mother Nature, instead of the instant and processed foods they eat now, we are helping them to return to a more natural way of living. By encouraging movement every day, we help them to create strong, healthy active bodies. These changes will help them to achieve better health and are better for the planet and generations to come.

As promised in the beginning, I have tried to fill this book with easy-to-understand information, tips, and suggestions that you can implement right away. If you like the book, please do me a favour and put a good review where you bought it. The greater the number of good reviews, the more the book is shown online and the more families I can help.

Finally, I want to give you a big shoutout. I know you are a busy parent with a lot going on, but you took the time to read the entire book. I hope I was able to give you the information that you were looking for in a way that resonated with you. Good luck on your health journey!